TUINA Baby Massage

中 国 推 拿

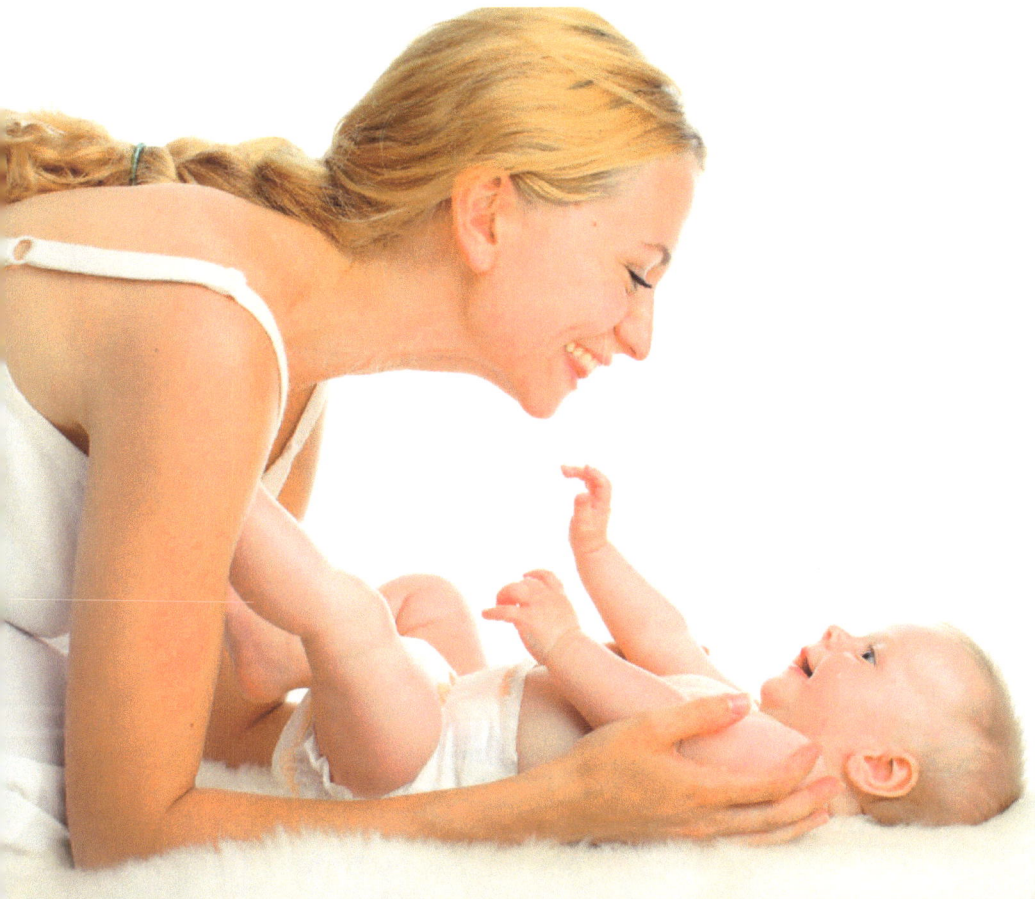

By Linda Larson

TUINA Baby Massage

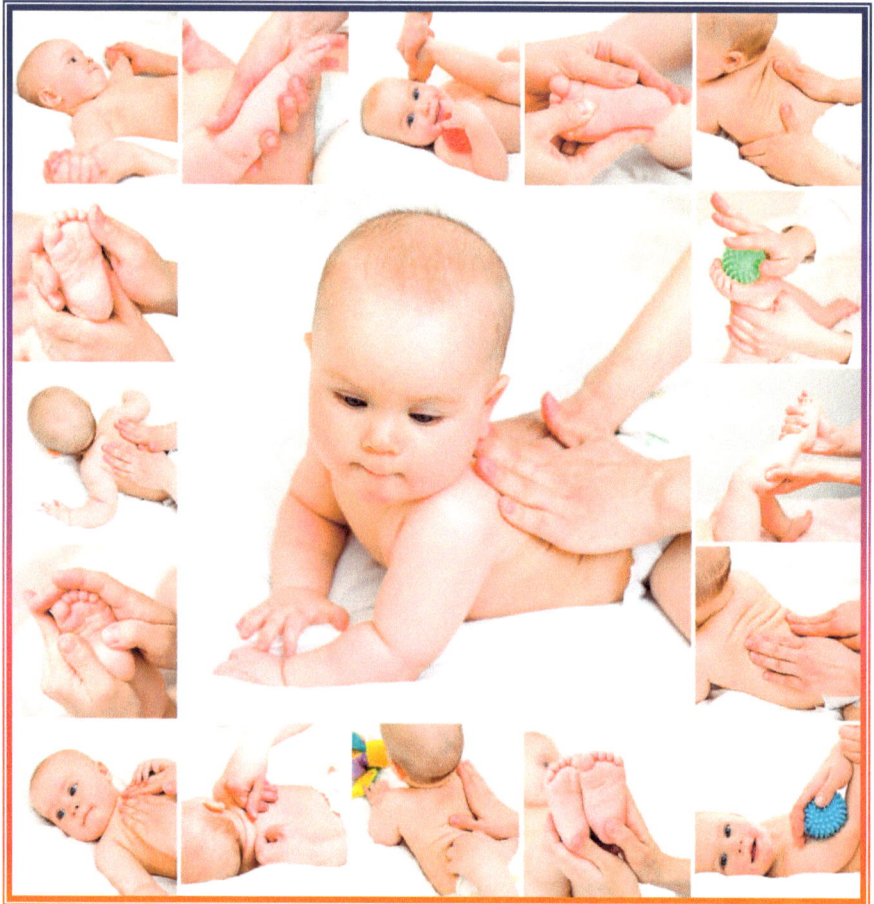

The New Mother's Guide Book where you will find
Massage Techniques for Every Baby's Delight

TUINA Baby Massage

By Linda Larson

ISBN: 978-0-9917470-7-8

www.Fae-Entertainment.ca

An Introduction to Baby Massage

*T*he Jiang-Su Provincial Hospital of Nanjing, China has a foundation main-stream medicine practice combined with Traditional Chinese Medicir Here a greater understanding of the human body and its functions are approach with complete balance, the best of both worlds in health care. In the Pediat Division at the Jiang-Su Provincial Hospital, health care is an issue because the are so many people in China's population to care for. Holistic or Ancient Chine Medicine is often less costly to the public than mainstream medical treatment. It a very efficient way for the medical care system to operate in China, using mc of the old ways to treat the body in health and disease through a main Provin Hospital. Taking care of a baby with special medical or health needs can becor challenging for a parent. In Chinese Traditional Medicine, a baby under physician's care may have Chinese Tuina Massage as a main treatment for t more mild medical symptoms, such as colic and a main-stream medical plan f the more diagnosed severe cases.

Currently, Chinese "Tuina" Massage is found as a main health-care regime more than 75 percent of young infants' medical care cases in China. This amazing to me, and one can only imagine just how many massages sever million children and adults receive in China every day. Tuina — Chine Massage is now being introduced to the outside world. China was not alwa open to the out-side world for any type entry into their world. I felt very lucky be included in our study group with the best Pediatric Division in China. I met woman having a small box lunch outside the Hospital grounds. She was studyi at Jiang-Su, researching cancer for John Hopkins. She said the doctors' skills this medical facility are a rarity in our world. My doctor and teacher, Dr. Y Ming, head of the Pediatric Division, was a little dainty woman about five fe one inch tall. She had great compassion for the infants and children that came her for treatment. Dr. Ming had studied in her home country to become a Medic Doctor, Acupuncturist, and then specialized in Pediatric Tuina - Chinese massa; for small children.

r. Ming's daughter accompanied her by translating Chinese medical text into nglish, so we could understand her better. Learning from the other doctors in the inics at The Jiang-Su Provincial Hospital was much more of a practical hands-1 treatment. We would learn through direct contact with babies and mothers. ven after spending the time learning the Holistic Chinese Medicine approach, I el there is still so much to learn from their ancient ways. The Chinese base all edical treatment with the function of the elements in nature. Heaven, earth, and e elements found in the body are the tools for which they diagnose and treat mptoms. How these elements are in balance with one another in the human)dy will often determine the outcome of focused treatment.

good massage provides relaxation, and often relief from pain, such as colic hen applied properly. It is always a good idea to determine the general health of baby through a mainstream doctor before beginning any massage or holistic erapy, should there be a contra-indication for the direct application. Massage is)t a replacement for mainstream medicine. For example, you would use ainstream medicine when you have a broken bone and would need an X-ray and cast. However, when your baby has "colic", a massage with Aromatherapy for e digestion may be just what the Doctor ordered.

uina Acupressure Massage and Aromatherapy is a complement to help the body ?al itself in an alternative form." - Linda Larson

4

Chapter 2
What you will need for your Baby's Massage

- Aromatherapy oil(s) or non-scented lotion

- Music source: Tape or CD player to play soft, soothing music

- One or two extra diapers on hand, just in case

- Stuffed animals, or soft squeezable toys

- Baby's sleeper with blanket for dressing after a baby's massage

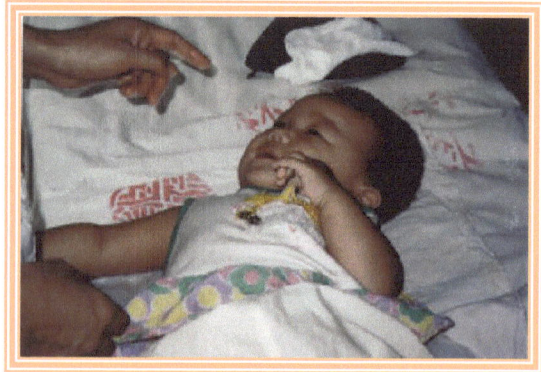

Setting up the massage space

- Warm to moderate room temperature

- Soft, muted lighting for baby's sensitive eyes and to promote calmness

- Flat surface to set massage oil/lotion or cream for stability purposes

- A flat, safe area for your baby to receive a massage, such as the floor, a futon or changing table

It's as easy as 1-2-3!

1.) Begin by placing the towel on the flat surface where your baby will be positioned for the massage.

2.) Protect the surface (such as carpeting or other) from spilling the oil/lotion or cream by always placing the bottle on the towel. Make sure the container is out of reach of your child's hands-they are very busy moving all the time!

3.) Start your music; play with the toys for awhile, and being by following the instructions for baby massage.

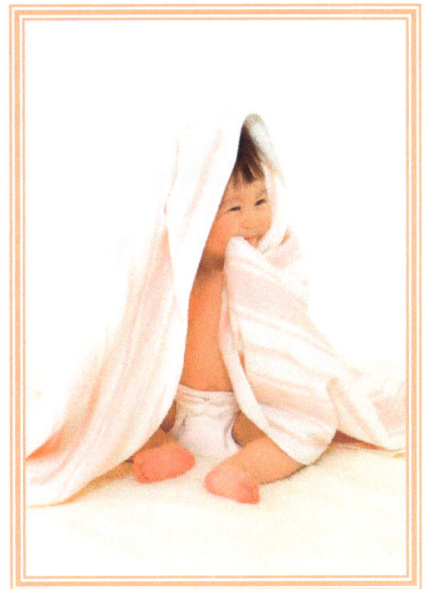

Best times for Baby's Massage

Time needed: Usually 20-35 minutes

- When baby has digestive pain

- Before nap time

- After baby's bath

- Before you have an important quiet time for yourself, a special event or before the baby sitter arrives
  - Anytime is a good time!

Massage and Human Touch

*M*assage and human touch have a common thread globally. Throughout histo[r]
one at-tribute most people seem to have is the need to give and receive love, and

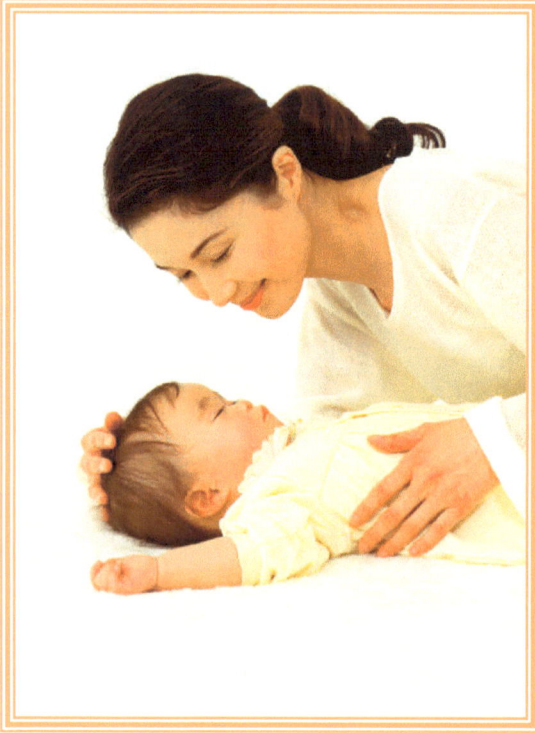

nurture and care for other human bein[g]
— especially our own family. The de[ep]
inner drive from Mother Nature sets t[he]
stage for human need to nest a[nd]
procreate. Before a baby is conceive[d]
there is physical contact oft[en]
accompanied by love between parents.

With the physical contact between m[an]
and woman meeting in the act of lo[ve]
intimacy and touch, a child is born. Af[ter]
birth, the instinctive survival mechanis[m]
is a need for physical connection to t[he]
parent figures. Touch creates hum[an]
emotions and feelings.

In "The Little Baby Massage Book[,"]
the goal is to help you create the mo[st]
nurturing, loving, caring and f[un]
environment for your baby! Massage c[an]
become an integral part of your life f[or]
years to come. Parents who have learn[ed]
how to give their baby a massage oft[en]
say just how wonderful it is for us to receive massage back from their children as th[ey]
grow! The after-effects of massage seem to live on in our children. Parents comme[nt]
when they come home after a hard day of work that they find their children eager to gi[ve]
a foot massage, a relaxing shoulder massage, accompanied by tickling, giggling, a[nd]
laughter. Parents often tell me how glad they were to have learned how to establi[sh]
positive touch, communication, and to give their children pediatric massage. *"The body [is]
a supreme temple of transformation, the place where all the forces of the universe gath[er]
to be channeled and transformed into a higher integral order of nature and spirit."*
By ~ Jean Houston

7

Bonding with your child

*B*onding with your child can become one of the most important activities in your relationship. Touch establishes a parent-child trust. Scientists have conducted research which confirms how important touch is. Infants and children cannot survive without human touch. Infants may develop a syndrome called Failure to Thrive. Research suggests that this syndrome may be linked to a lack of love and human touch. The symptoms suggest the infants have an inability to digest, assimilate, and absorb nutrients into their body properly.

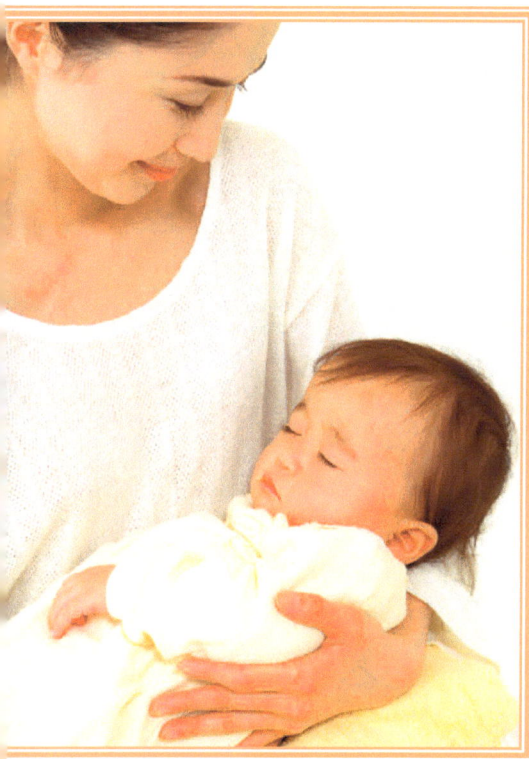

Weight loss is very common with Failure to Thrive Syndrome (or commonly called Infantile Anorexia), and infants have been put on special massage, nutrition, and personal contact schedules while being treated by the proper medical professionals. In adults, this syndrome may be medically referred to as Anorexia.

Massage just plain feels good! Even with all that scientific data, proof, and research. Documenting what massage does in the human body is great, but a more simple way to say it would be; human caring.

In the medical research, we see clearly that infants need caring touch, nurturing, emotional support, and love on a regular basis in order to remain healthy. Infants are under just as much stress as adults.

touch is thought to be more positive, children may be more likely to have less shame about their body. Massage can help to build better self-esteem, a stronger immune system, better memory retention, and trust in parental authority figures.

A Quick Meditation for Parents

*I*magine … floating, laughing, and playing together. Then hug! When you hug your child, you are also hugging yourself.

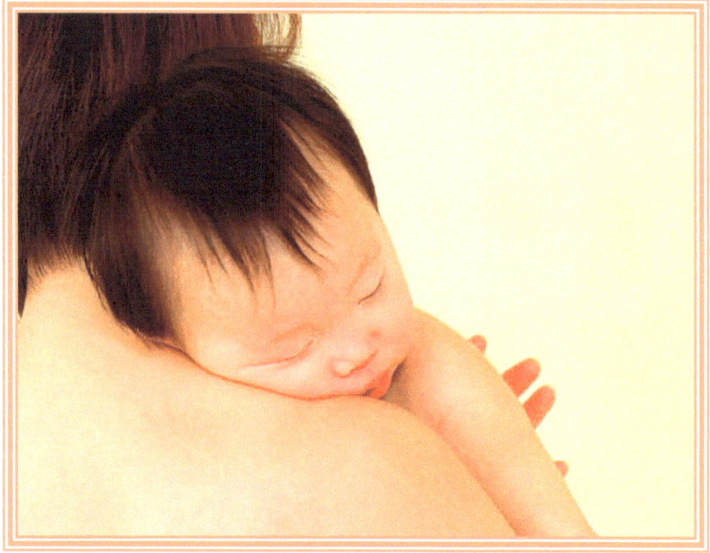

Close your eyes…
Hold your child close to your heart
Visualize having a heart as big as Mother Earth
Imagine the most beautiful sky blue you can dream
Breathe slowly in through your nose, and out through your mouth
Begin breathing silently in the words "Love and Joy"
Breathe out silently the words, "Peace and Harmony"
After you establish a slow peaceful breath, begin breathing out
With "Peace and Harmony" blowing pink bubbles!

Continue the meditation if you like it and eventually see yourself and your child encased in one very large pink bubble. This meditation was designed for those who want to give their children the gift of love and trust.

1-2-3 Meditation
For New Mothers

Close your eyes, breathe deeply, slowly, silently say to yourself;

    1) I see my child whole, healthy and complete
            (rub your tummy gently)

    2) I am a whole, healthy and complete mother

    3) Breathe in … and simply say, **"I AM LOVE"**
       (Imagine a big rainbow heart around you)

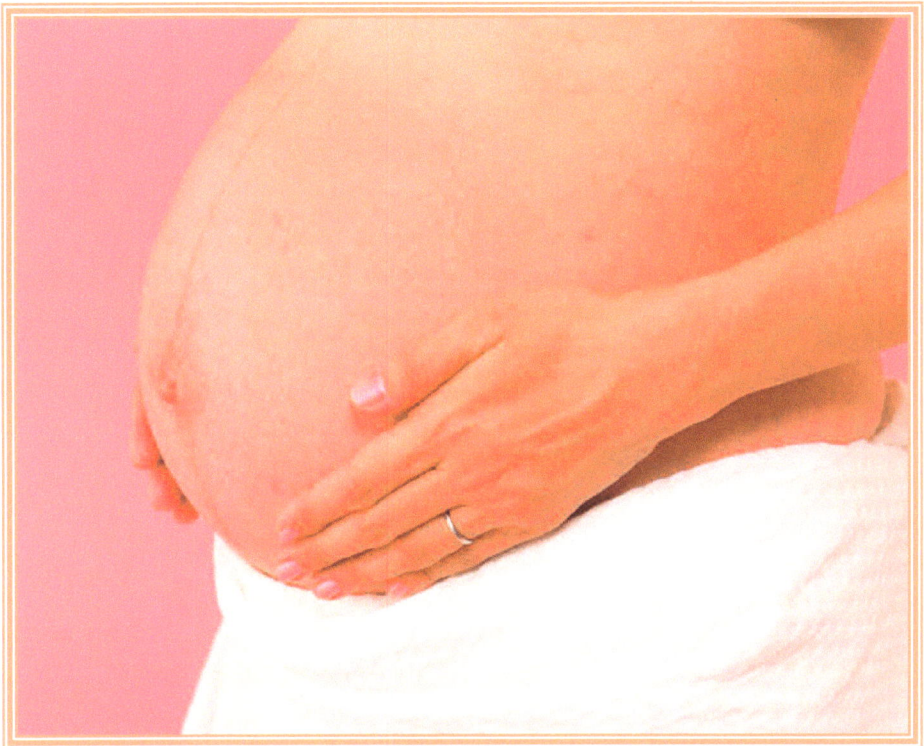

"Mommy Meditation"

If one finds that becoming a new mom is stressful, this might help ...

• Sit, lay down, find a comfortable position to relax and close your eyes

• Breathe slowly, deeply, Silently repeat to yourself;

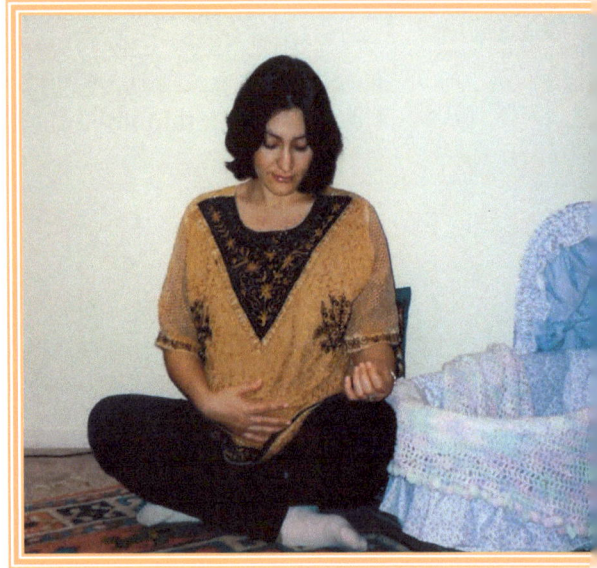

My body is light
I am calm and bright
My mind is clear
I have no fear
It is easy to love
I receive my energy
From Love and Light
I am filled with Blessings
Freedom
Peace and Harmony

Use the color green for this meditation, visualizing for peace and harmony. Newness is often felt with the color green. Green grass, a green piece of clothing, a green candle, or flowers with green in them works wonders throughout your day after this meditation is complete. Go for a walk with your baby today, and look the green trees, grass ... nature in a local park.

A the **Nordstrom Medical Tower in Seattle, WA., U.S.A.**, infants born with substance addiction appeared to benefit from massage. Infants are not programmed to believe that massage does or does not work. Here it was discovered that massage increases ACTH production.* the body can respond to massage, touch and love biochemically healing itself.

ACTH: Adrenocortocotrophic Hormone – Is released through the master pituitary gland. ACTH being released into the endocrine system helps the central nervous system slow down long enough to taper off convulsions or withdrawals to substance additions. The immune system is then stimulated by the secretions of the endocrine system.

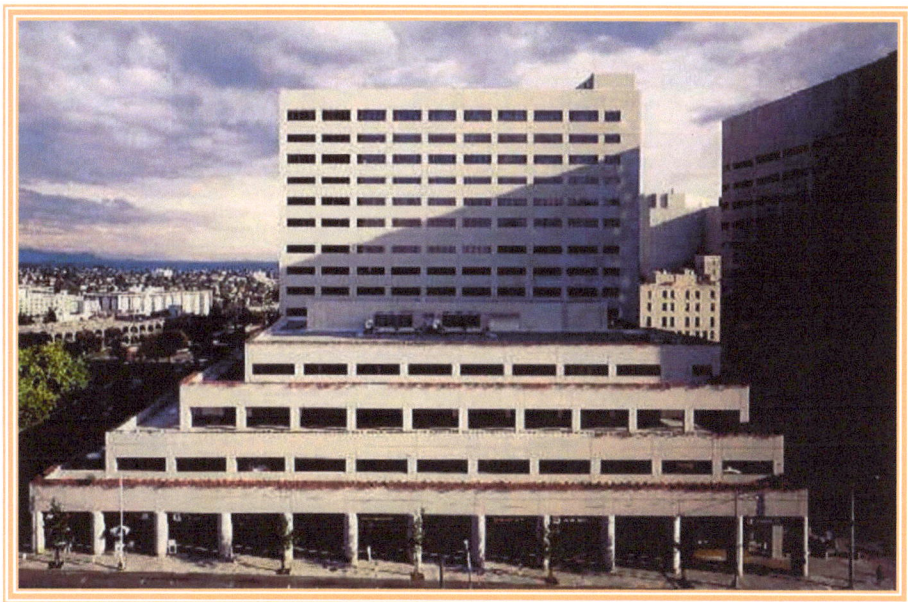

Nordstrom Medical Tower
Seattle, WA., U.S.A.

Chapter 5
How To Massage Hand Techniques

1) Circular friction using the finger tips and thumbs

2) Flat fingers and palm down (for circular friction or effleurage)

3) Acupressure with the thumb (using the thumb pad)

4) Thumb acupressure while bracing the thumb with fingers (ideal for shoulders, neck and back, etc.)

5) Direct acupressure with index finger (pressure is applied with the pad of the index finger.)

Note: Fingernails should be clipped, short, and filed to avoid injury while applying massage movements.

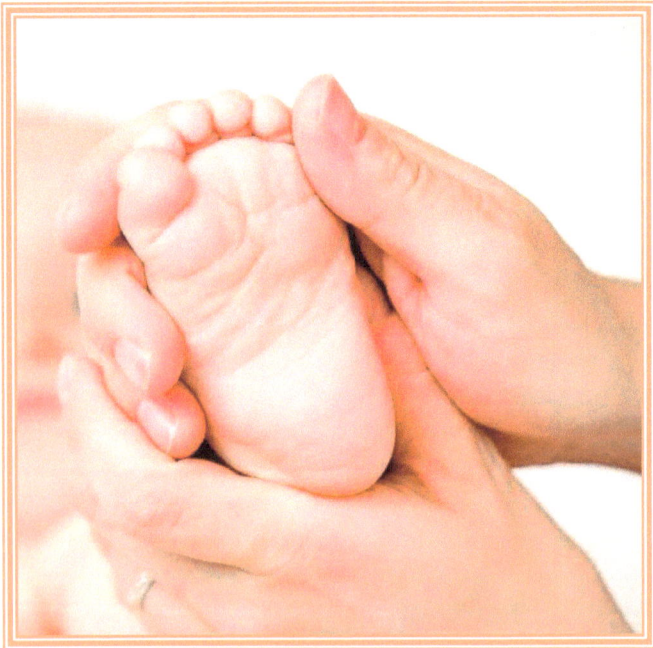

"Neibagua Fulling"
Hand Massage and Fulling

...lling is easy and gentle. Take the palm of your hands together, and begin in the ...nter of the baby's palm, working outwards toward the little pinkies (smallest ...gers).

...) Neibagua fulling or clockwise massage is good for digestive relief and colic.

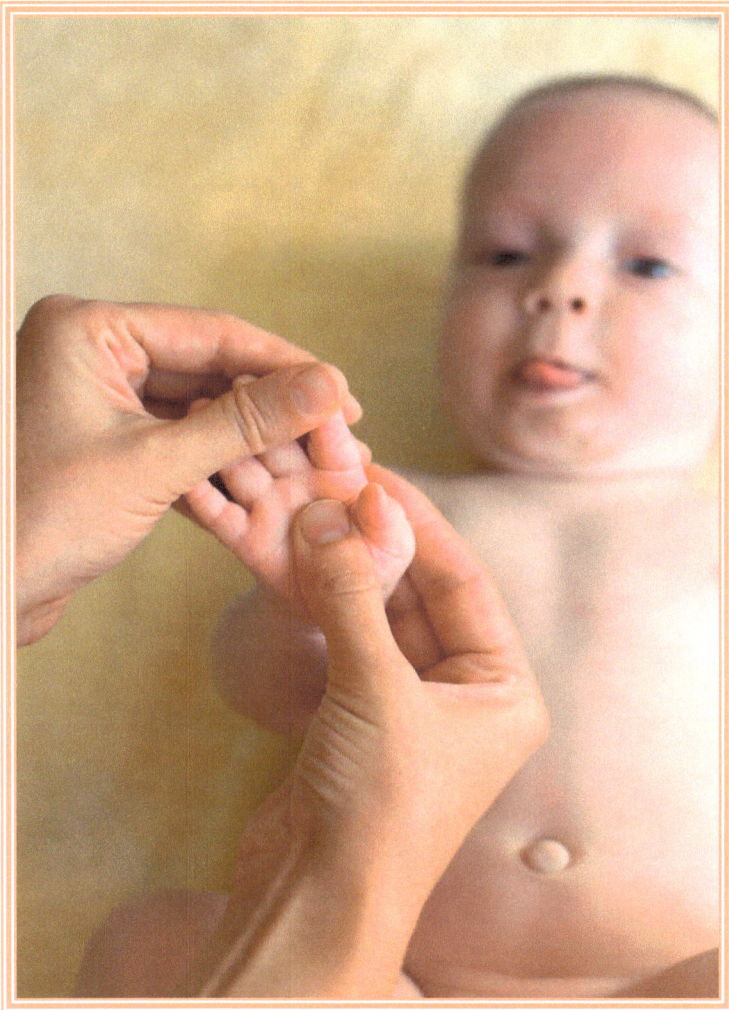

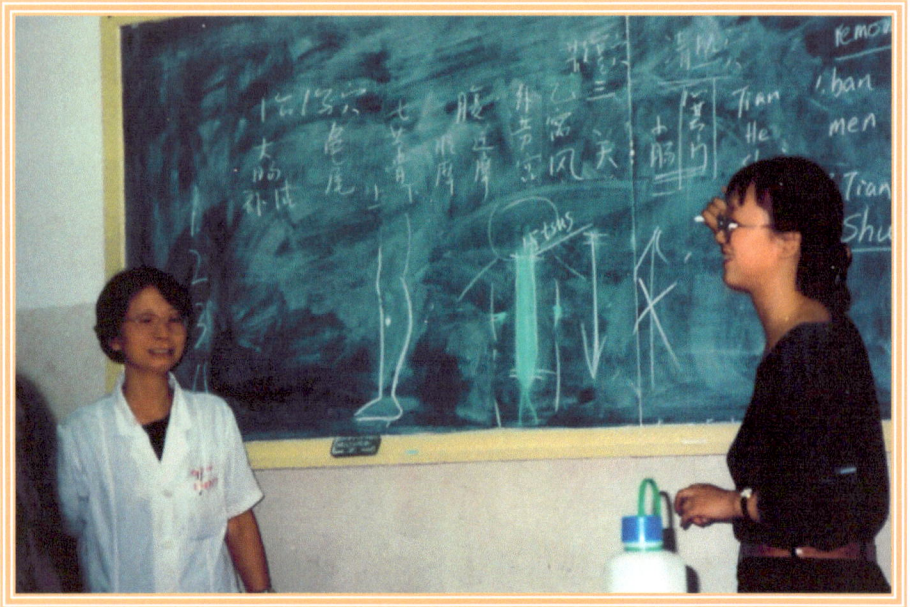

"Neibagua Massage –
Around and around in a
circle, rotating clockwise,
the palm of your hand,
the center of the universe."

Dr. Yin Ming
Pediatrics at Nanjing, China

"Renzhong"

Acupressure point for "Balance"

1) Press lightly underneath the nose in the indent just above the upper lip for 30 seconds up to two minutes.

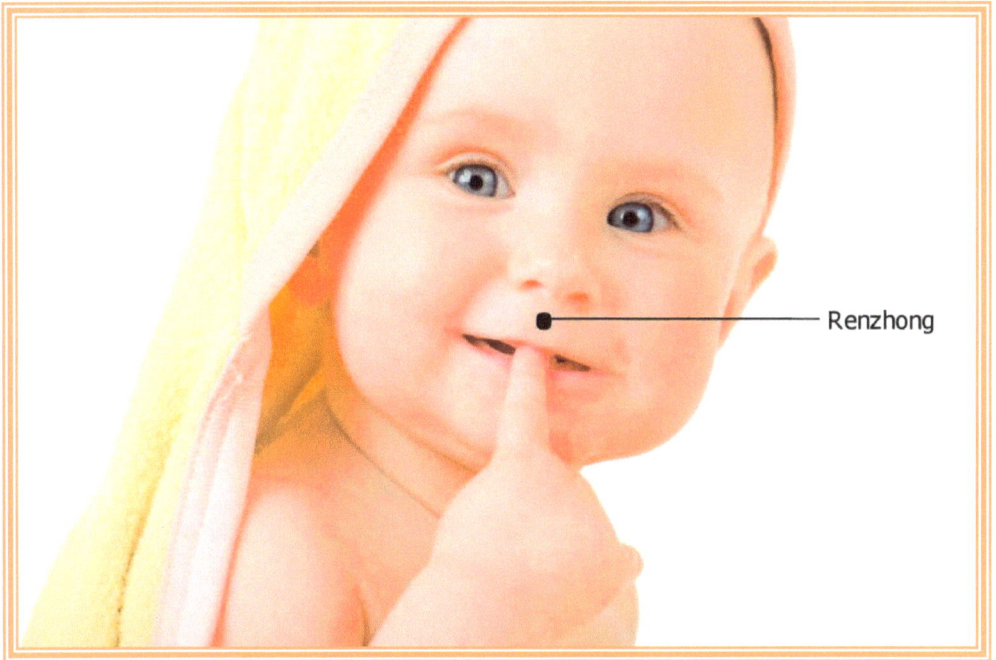

Renzhong

Renzhong is the "main" acupressure point in the body

is used to regain the ability of inner peace, balance, regaining vision of the eyes, and lming an otherwise traumatic reaction that may have occurred during a serious fall, cident, or near death experience. It can also stop "seizures" and crying "fits." The inese call this the Point of Balance.

"Digestive Relief"

*W*hen your baby has colic, a massage can help them feel more comfortabl

during such a painful tummy time. Of course the symptoms can be congestio
fever, aches, gas, bloating and feeling restless. Crying is the only way to let yo
know they hurt. If there is any health concern, please consult your family docto
for the use of massage. This is not a medical replacement treatment - massage ju
feels good!

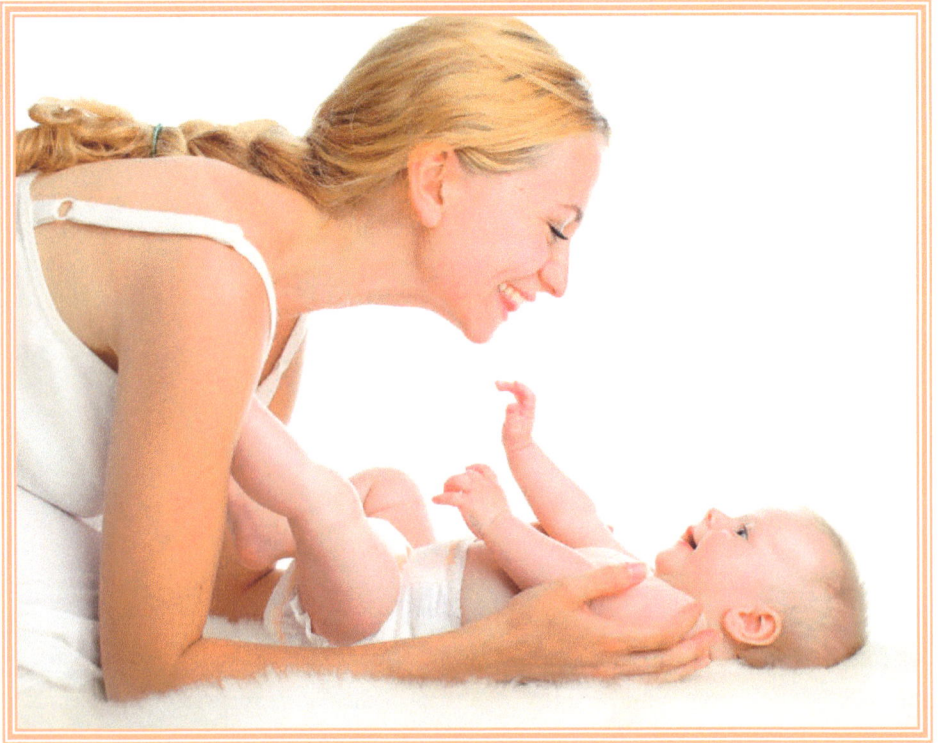

"Fulling"

$\mathcal{F}$ulling is used to introduce your touch, apply oil/lotion to the skin, warm the

sue, and increase circulation. In Swedish Massage techniques, it is important to rm up the area before going in deeper, lessening pain as well as the promotion trust in the person giving massage to another. Just as when you exercise, you st stretch and warm muscles before and after exercise; Massage is based on the ne principle. Note: Always make sure your hands are warm before applying -lotion to the skin directly.

Start by applying a small amount of massage oil or lotion to the palms of your nds.

"Tanzong" — Begin the massage in the middle of the baby's chest/tummy :a, hands flat, applying very light pressure.

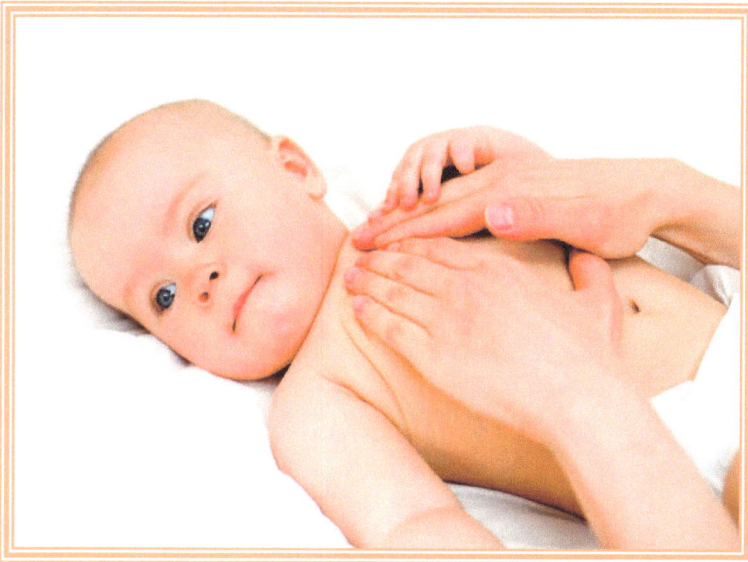

3) "Fu Yin-Yang" — Smoothly begin to part the hands outward to the sides of the baby's body

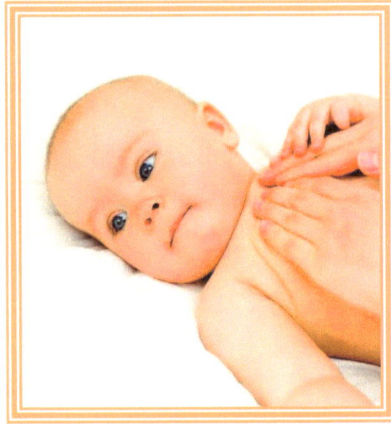

4) Finally the hands sweep gently to the sides of the baby's body; lift the hands off, and start again from the middle of the chest/tummy area.

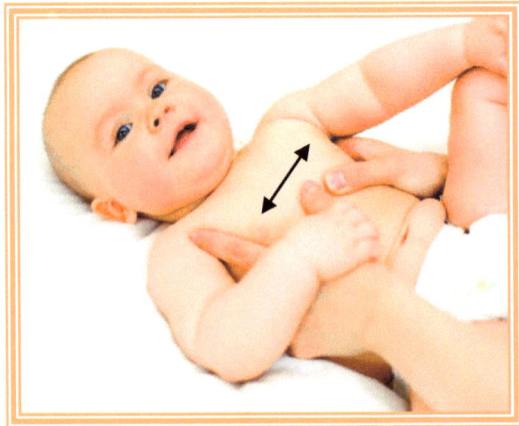

Note: Repeat fulling 3, 5 or 7 times until you feel the baby is warm and accustomed to your touch (this i great time to tickle baby a little bit). Re-apply massage oil or lotion if skin has absorbed the amount y used. Don't stop, keep massaging! In massage education, the teachers all say, never lose contact with y massage subject. It will continue to establish trust if you practice this continuously. Once you become a p it will be so much fun! Soft music in the background is great to help keep the massage relaxing and f easier. Try to remember to start playing the music before you apply oil or lotion to your hands, or it will all over the stereo!

"Circular Movement"

iagram for "Digestive Relief"

) Kneading "Dantian" - Use one hand with flat extended fingers, and apply a ght, circular clock-wise movement to the abdomen.

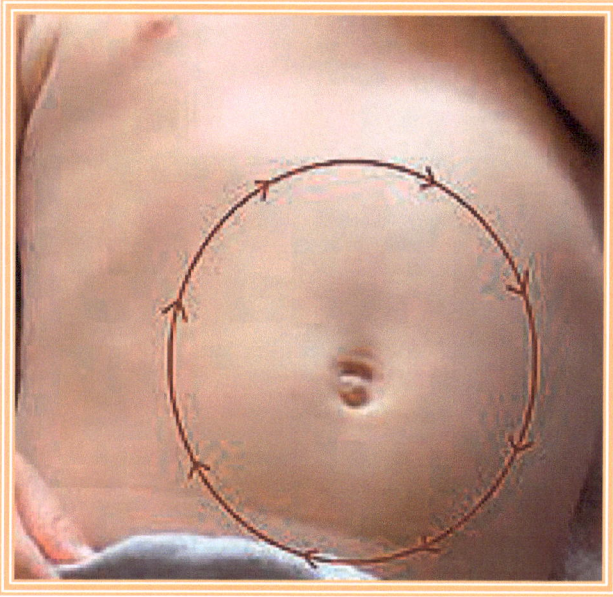

Make sure your fingers stay under the rib cage, and above the fold in the legs. his is the area of "digestive relief." If your baby is uncomfortable, bring them in upright position, pat the upper back gently while they are over your shoulder tomach facing you).

3) Apply this massage technique three times for relaxation, five times for digestive pain, and seven times for more sever gaseous symptoms/constipation/colic disorders.

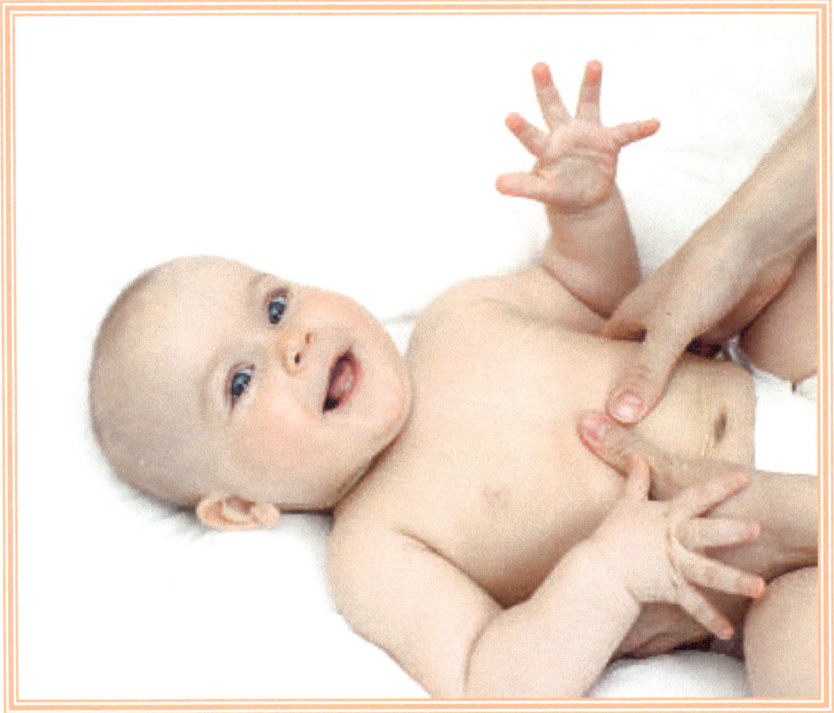

4) Apply more oil/lotion if needed, to keep baby's skin smooth, soft and easy for gliding your hand through the massage.

Note: This massage technique is a great way to get the digestive flow moving and flowing. Make sure your baby has their diaper on before you continue, or you might find something unexpected!

"Dujiao" Acupressure Point
For Digestive Relief and Colic

"Dujiao" - With your index finger, thumb, or middle finger apply light pressure the abdomen as shown in detailed diagram/illustration.

Measure one inch over to the right of baby's belly button, and one inch down wards the lower abdomen (facing you it would be to your left).

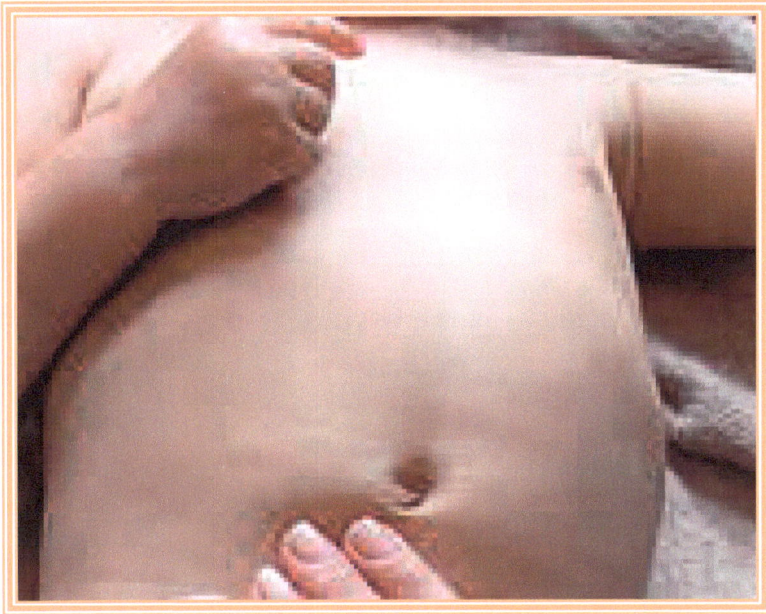

Apply pressure gently to the lower abdomen for approximately 30 seconds, up 90 seconds for more painful digestive colic disorders.

Repeat circular movement technique after this acupressure point has been plied for 3x-5x.

Gastric and Peristalsis Observation
Massage Studies

A the **Qingdao Medical College, Shandong Province,** with th

assistance of the **Tuina Therapy Department,** "Massage experiments als
showed that increased gastric digestion was seen after manipulations on the poin
to reinforce the spleen, and y far more increased gastric digestion was found whe
manipulations had been applied to the points strengthening the spleen and to th
Neibagua point."

The Massage experiments prove that Tuina therapy may motivate the conveyir
of the meridians (acupressure point lines) and cure diseases.

(Neibagua acupressure point definition and location: Neibagua is found in th
center of the palm of the hand. Its functions are to reinforce the spleen, increas
digestion movement in a more calming way.)

Luan Changye
Beijing, China
Infantile Tuina Therapy

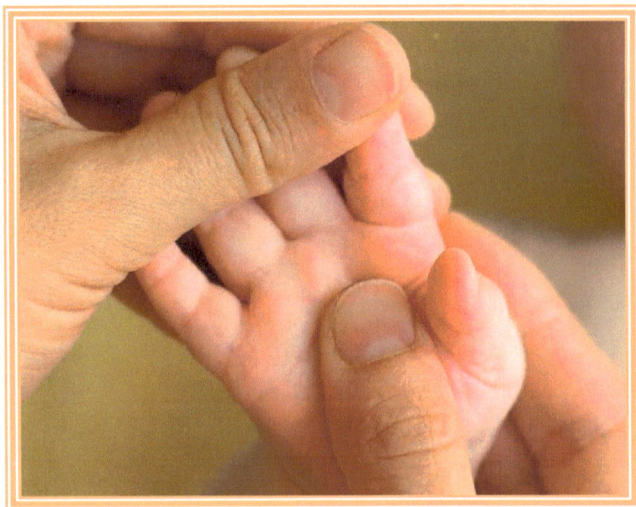

Draw with your fingers on baby's tummy;

I Love U!

In the shape of a heart…

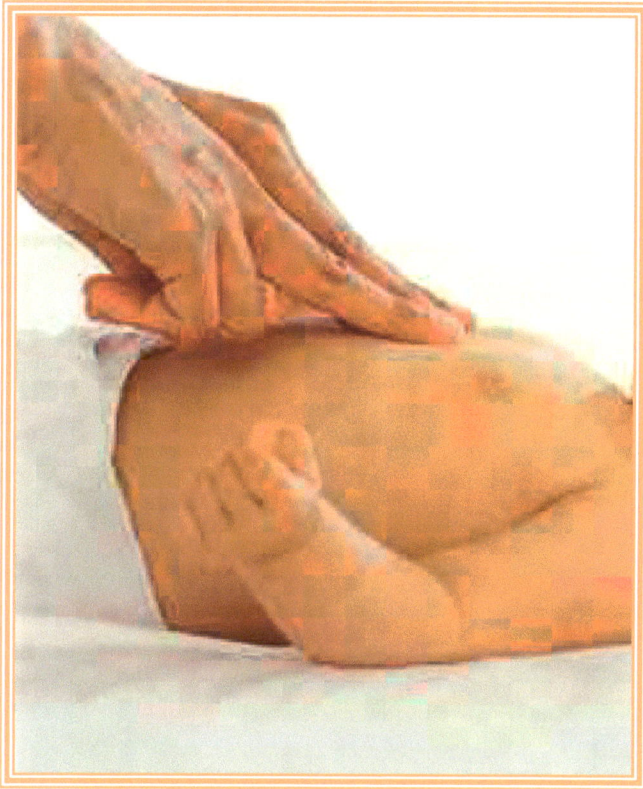

Tummy massage makes baby feel so much better!

"Cradle the ankles" Movement

1) Firmly (but not too tightly) hold the ankles together with bracing both legs.

2) Lift lower part of the baby's body while baby lays on their back.

3) Lift baby's bottom and spine "up" while keeping the spine completely straight.

*Refer to photo.

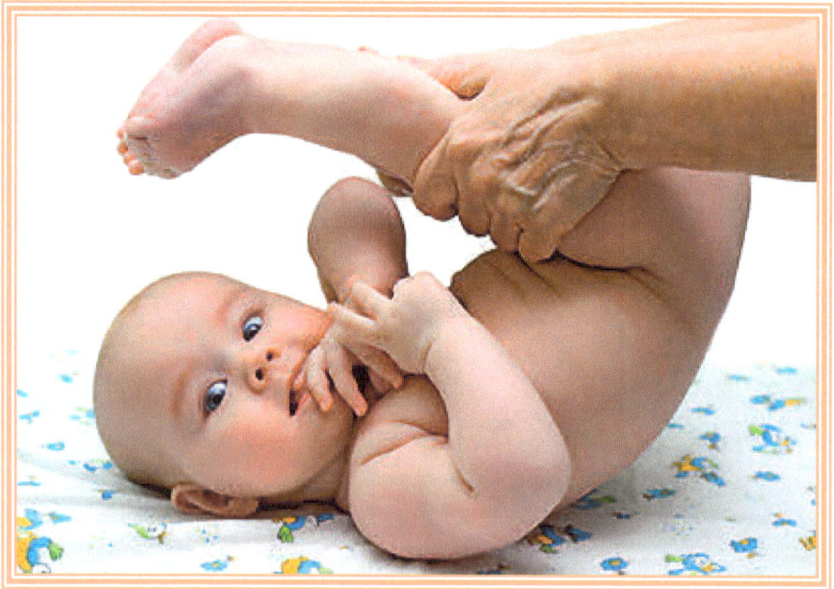

4) Bring the baby's feet towards its face (infants are very flexible) while holdin feet firmly, and hold for five seconds, then slowly bring baby back down to sam starting position. Again, gently while keeping baby's spine straight during th movement; no rocking the body back and forth.

"Cradle the Ankles" Movement

his is a great time to tickle, giggle, sing a song and pat the tummy! Enjoy your
ne, make it playful. Unless baby is sleepy - they may want it quiet too.

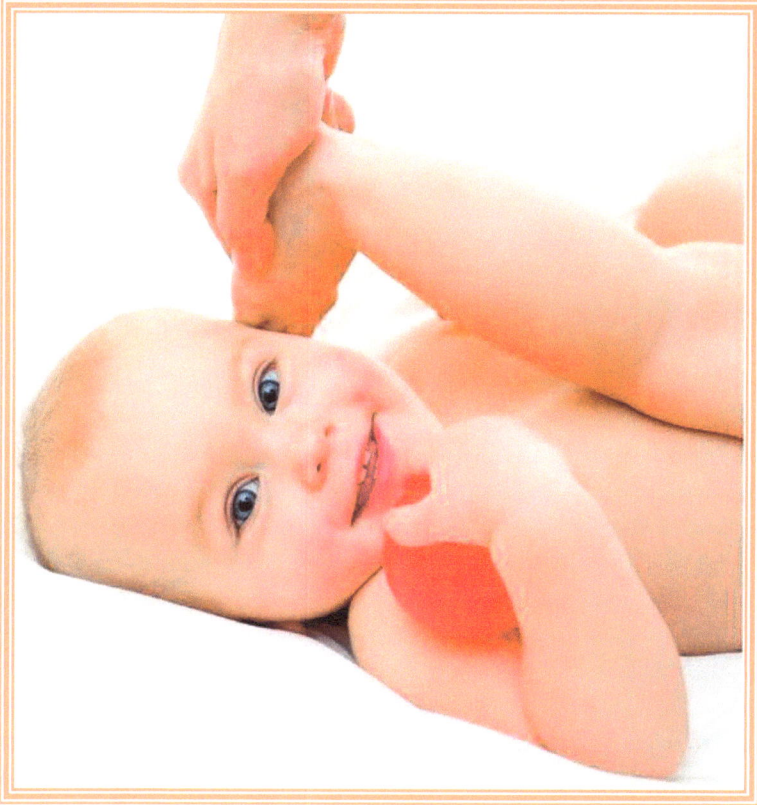

Repeat "Circular Movement" massage technique, and you can do one leg at a
ne if you like.

Repeat "Cradle the Ankles" movement again, one time. This may be done up to
·ee times.

"Pat your Baby's Back"

1) Pat your baby's back gently as you cradle them over your shoulder as they ma[y]
need to be "burped!" The digestion relief acupressure points and massage yo[ur]
baby has received may begin to relieve the trapped bubbles. This is the same wa[y]
you burp your baby after feeding time. Cover your shoulder with a soft cloth f[or]
baby, just in case.

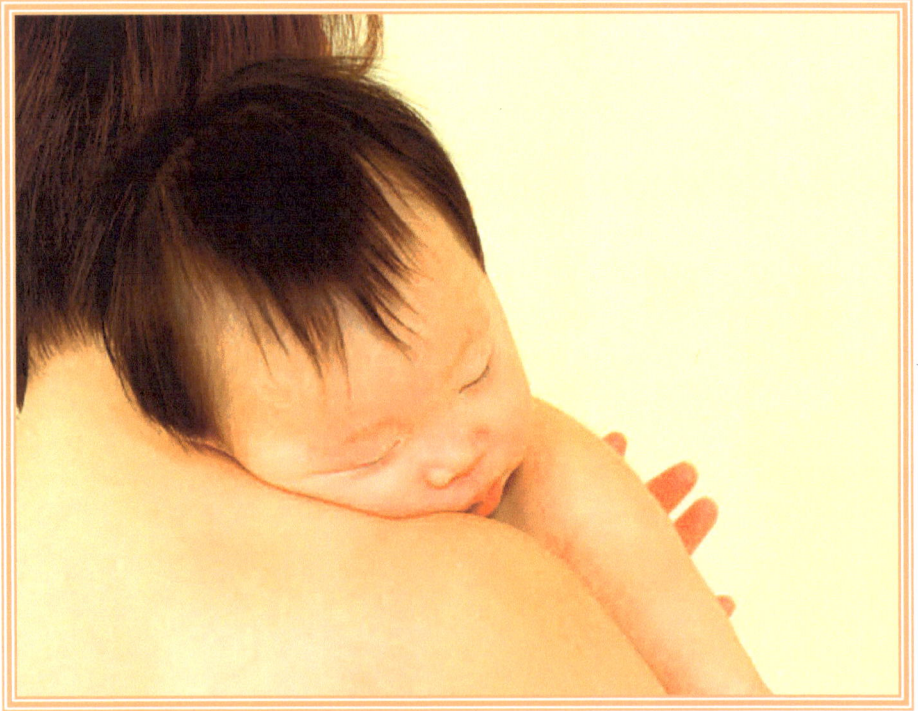

*Note: As you have baby in an upright position, fluids may begin movin[g]
through the digestive tract. Through basic gravity, the light pats help t[he]
assimilation and elimination of food, milk, or liquids. You can spend some ext[ra]
time with baby on your shoulder; rock baby back and forth. Much better!*

The "Arm Massage"
Indian Wringing Stretch (or milking)

Begin at the base of the arm (closest to baby's body).

Wring back and forth as you would milking or wringing out a wash cloth full water, starting from the base of the arm closest to the baby's body. Work your ay towards the elbow, wrist, and then lightly stretch the hand and fingers (a ntle movement).

Stretch your baby's palm with the flat of your hands together (like making a ncake). Start over again, repeat three to five times. Gently please!

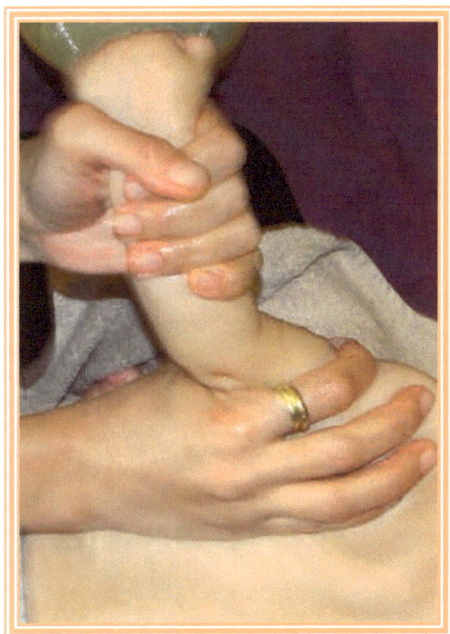

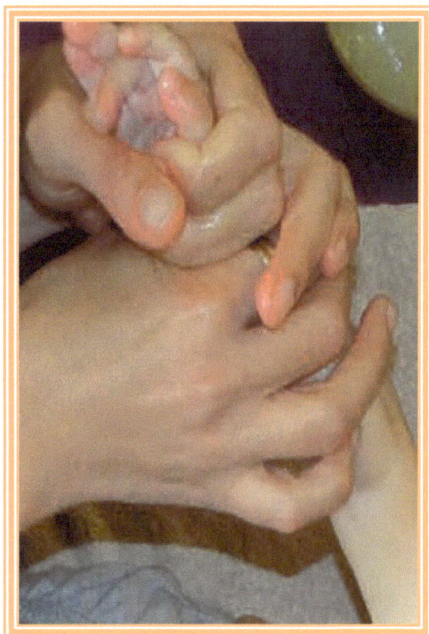

"Boyangchi Arm Massage"
Acupressure Point for Tummy Relief

1.) Apply a light index finger just lateral to elbow and one thumb print above the indentation for one minute.

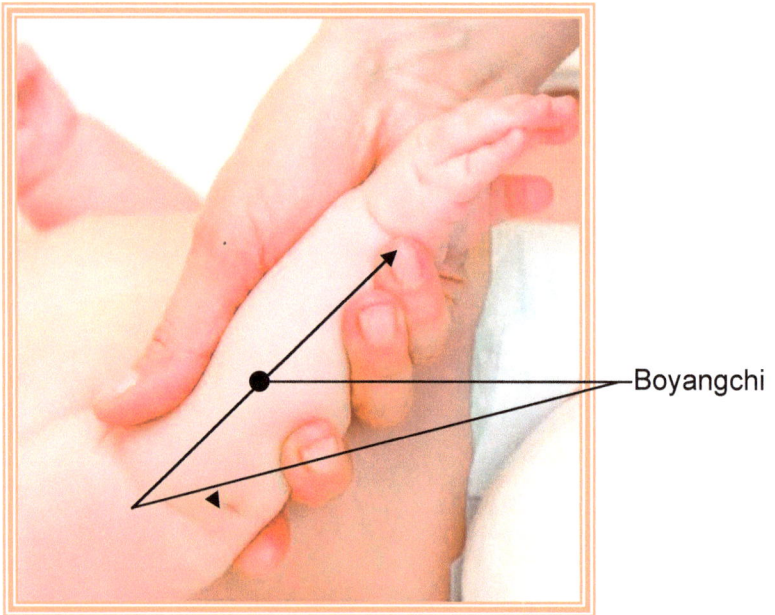

Boyangchi

2.) You may apply a gentle counter-clockwise movement with the same fing after the acupressure point has been held for one minute, gently stroke downwal to Boyangchi. Imagine using a broom to sweep a floor, a light sweeping motic with your finger.

Note: This is the yang dorsal acupressure point that can be done if your baby needs extra digestive relief (for increasing the yang energy).

"Tianheshui Arm Massage"
Acupressure Point for Fever Relief

1.) Apply a light index fingers medial to elbow half way above the wrist for up to one minute. This is a very soothing massage technique, and gets results quickly. Using a massage ball with light pressure (like the one in the photo) works really great too!

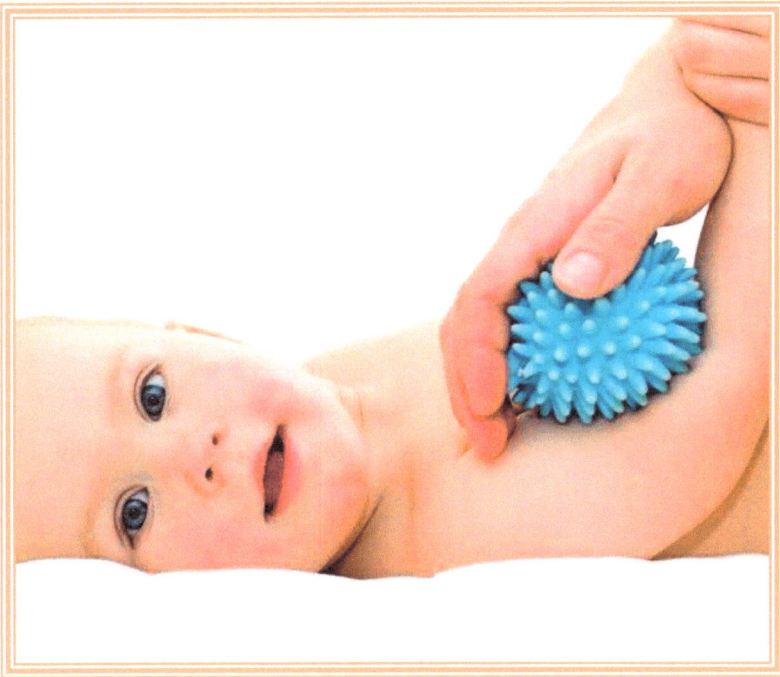

2.) With the same fingers after the acupressure point has been held for one minute, gently stroke upward to the small indent in elbow. Imagine using a broom to sweep a floor, a light sweeping motion with your finger. Gentle sweeping motions towards the heart. You can make this a little game; sing something like "Itsy, Bitsy Spider," or "Mary Had a Little Lamb!" This acupressure point that can be done if your baby has a common cold, abdominal pain, internal heat or fever symptoms (for decreasing heat energy).

"Indian Wringing" Leg Massage
Stretch (or milking)

1)   Start at the base of the leg (closest to baby's bottom).

A) Hold hands at the base of leg, and wring gently   B. Continue wringing,
   towards the feet

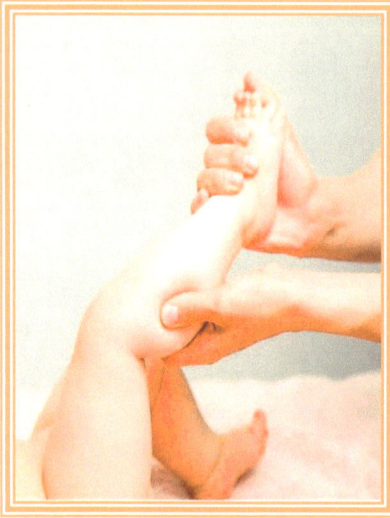

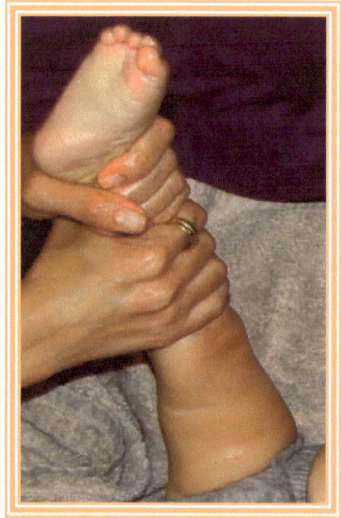

2) Wring back and forth while providing an easy stretch to the leg, working all the
way out to the little toes.

"Neck Massage"
(at the Occiput ridge of the skull)

There are two safe positions to apply these acupressure points while massaging fants under three years:

A) Baby facing you, being held in your lap with one arm wrapped around their back

B) Baby facing away held in your lap with one arm wrapped around their waist , or on a padded surface face down

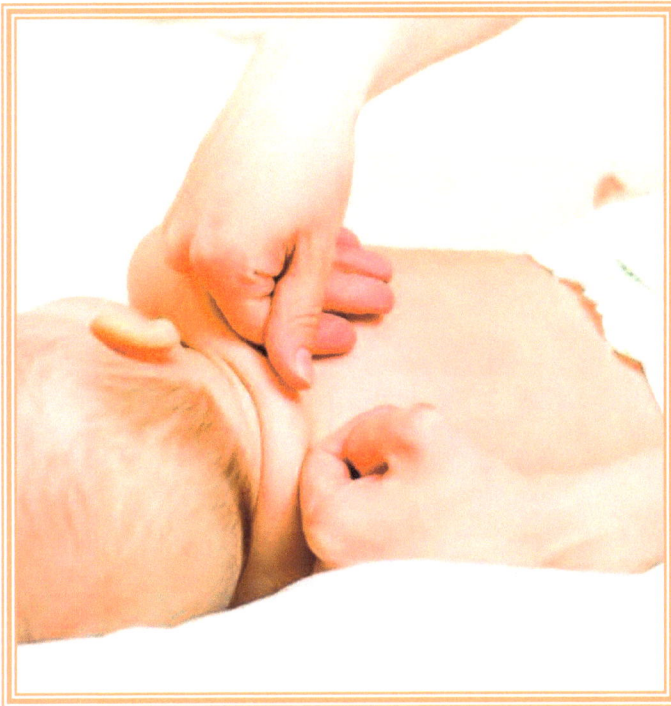

Begin by applying very light pressure and using "Circular" movement with the dex fingers and thumbs.

"Candy Cane Massage"
For the Back and Spine

PLEASE DO NOT PRESS DIRECTLY ON THE SPINE.
(Stay at least one half inch lateral to spine at all times.)
Be very careful to apply light pressure. The spine is not
fully developed in a young infant and may be sensitive.

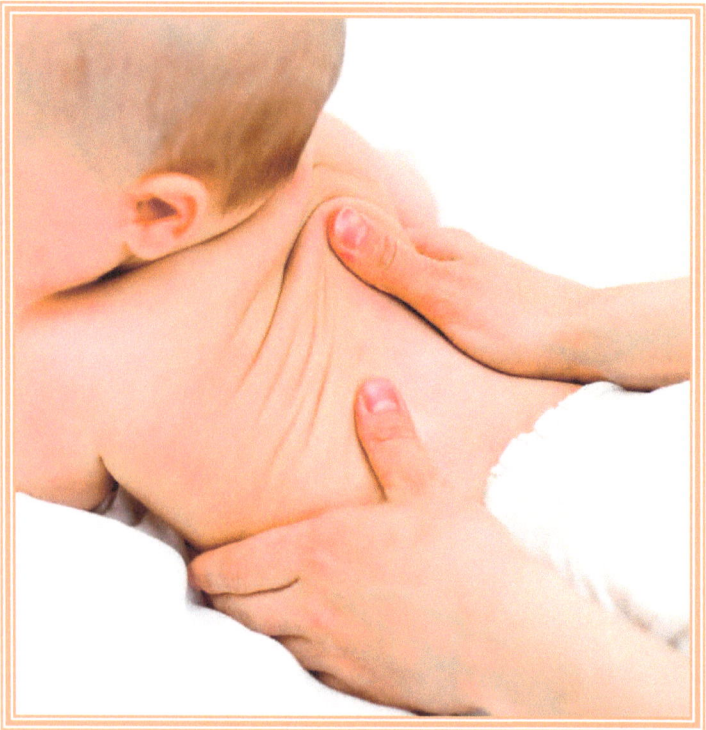

Note: If your baby exhibits any discomfort laying on their stomach, drape them over one shoulder and try the same back massage method while in an upright position (or, in some cases discontinue if baby is too fussy).

"Candy Cane Massage" Cont.
For the Back and Spine

There are three different body positions for your baby to relax in while you perform this massage movement;

      1) Baby can lay on their stomach, or face you

      A) A flat surface (soft floor/pillow)

      B) Draped over your legs

      C) Baby faces you in an upright position, laying over your shoulder comfortably

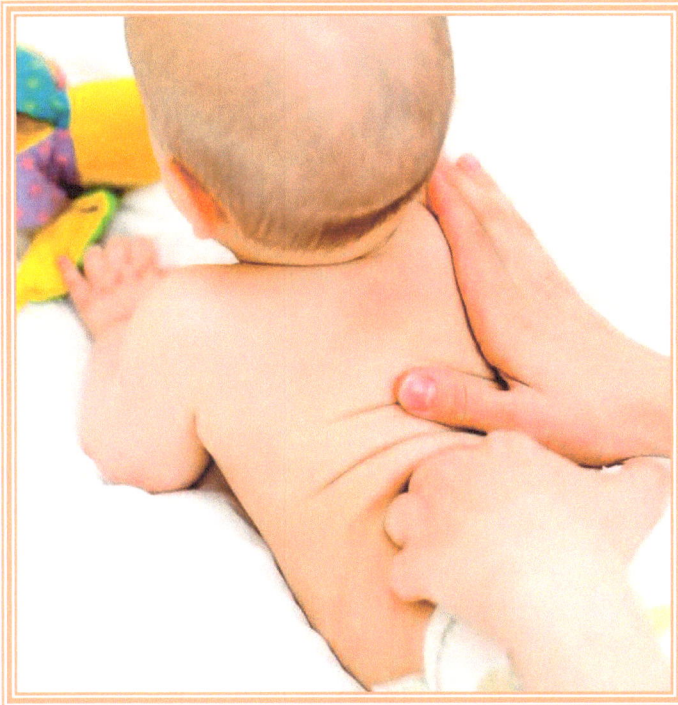

"Candy Cane Massage" Cont.
For the Back and Spine

2.) Baby laying on their tummy with pillow;

A) Using a pillow over your knee works great too!

(Make sure the baby's face can breathe at all times, and that they are completely comfortable.)

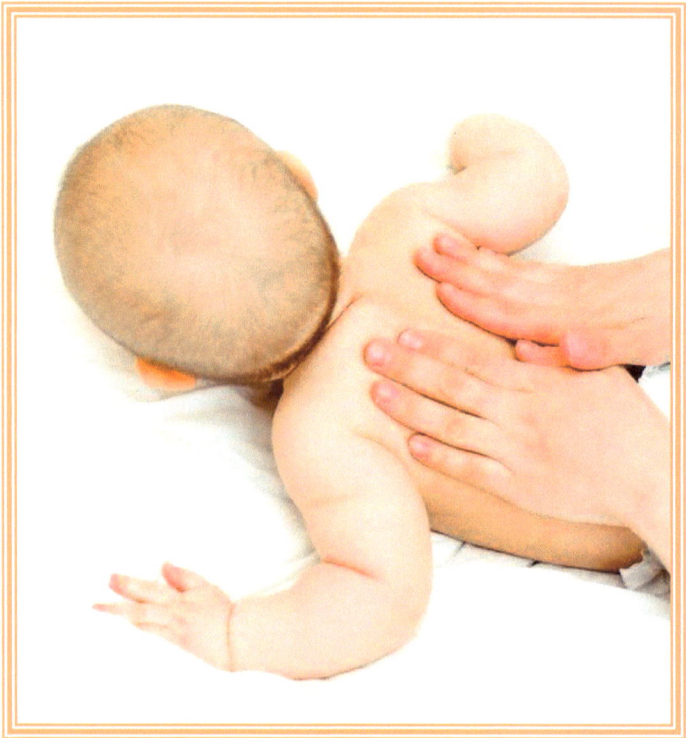

"Candy Cane Massage" Cont.
For the Back and Spine

Begin at the base of the spine (lower back) on the right or left side one-half
ch away from the spine.

With your thumb or finger, begin to massage in the shape of a candy cane (or
oside down J) staying at least one-half inch away from the spine. Please refer to
agram/illustration. Baby draped over legs while laying on tummy.

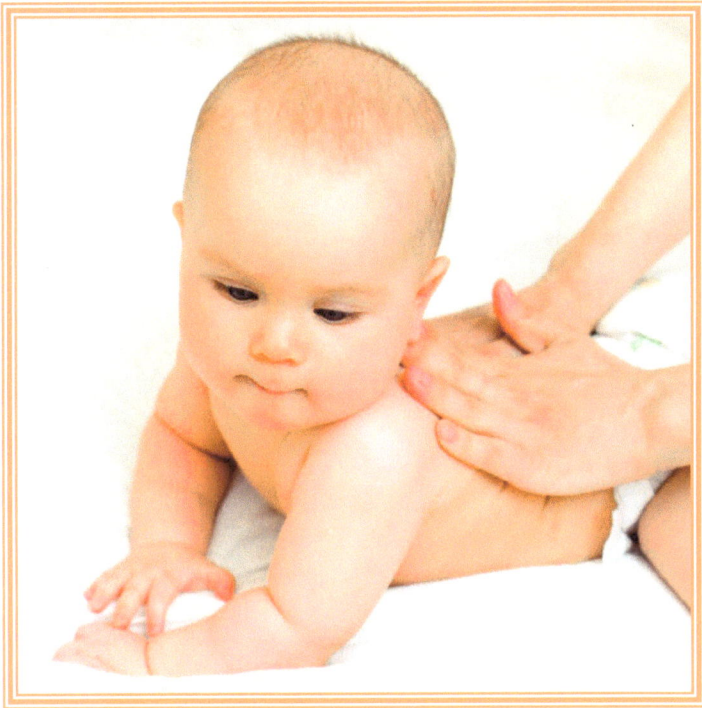

Seven to twelve "Candy Canes" can be drawn with your fingers all the way up
our baby's back to the nape of their little neck. The number of times you move
oward will depend on just how long the torso (upper body) is.

"Guwei Massage"

"Turtle's tail" Massage

Guwei – Tip of coccyx (tailbone) towards head, 17 massage strokes; Fc relief of diarrhea, dysentery, abdominal pain and prolapsed rectum Imagine using a broom to sweep a floor, a light sweeping motion wit your fingers.

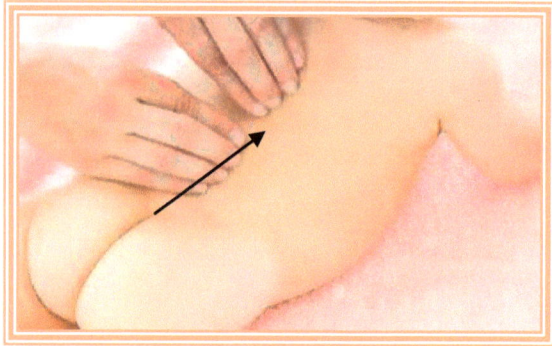

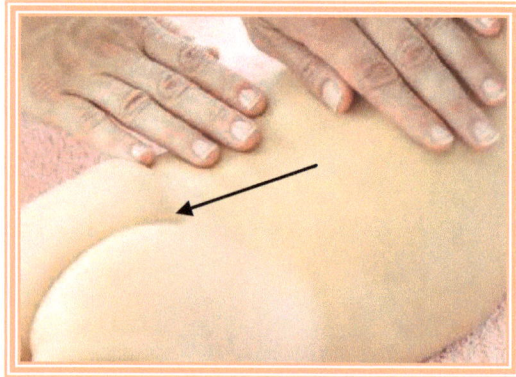

Guwei- Tip of coccyx (tailbone) toward feet, 17 massage strokes; Fc relief of constipation and poor (slow) digestion. Imagine using a broom t sweep a floor, a light sweeping motion with your finger.

"Skin Rolling"

There are two safely performed positions to utilize skin rolling.

A) Baby is facing you, sitting in your lap, held by one of your arms around their waist.

B) Baby is draped over your legs.

PLEASE, AVOID DIRECT PRESSURE ON THE SPINE

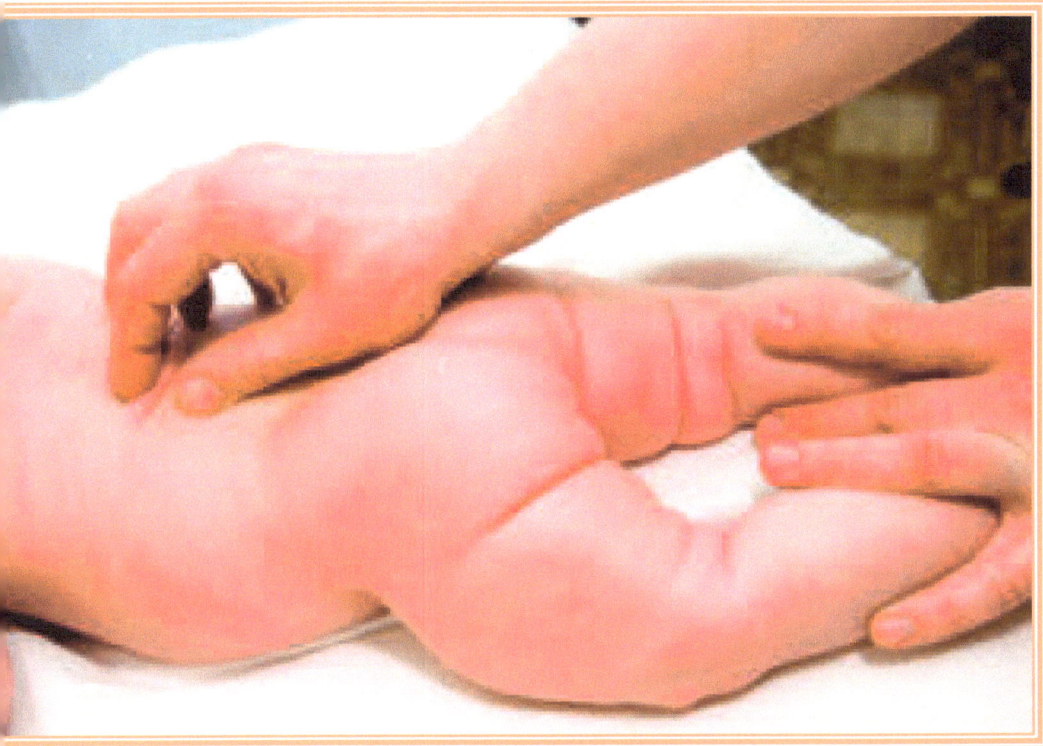

Infants should only receive the hand applied skin rolling technique
ONE-HALF INCH AWAY FROM THE SPINE

1) Begin at the lower spine, just **ONE-HALF INCH AWAY** from the spine. Begin skin rolling…

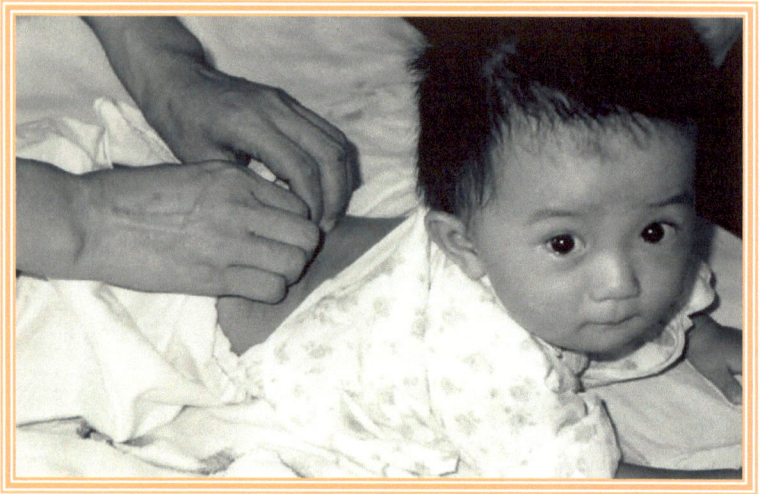

2) Pick up skin gently, and walk your fingers upwards, leaving the thumb as an anchor to follow. Repeat all the way up to the nape of the neck. Lightly Please! Baby's spine is their Central Nervous System area.

Thank you.

Baby Face Facial Massage
"Fulling the Forehead"

This is a very calming sedating massage movement. It is ideal before a nap. There are two positions for safe application:

A) Baby faces away from you while sitting in lap, a stable chair, or even a stroller. Ideal for cranky children while mom is out shopping. Or, directly in front of you, with back support such as; sitting in a stroller or propped up by a pillow. You can also gently place your baby on their back atop the changing table to apply this massage technique.

B) Laying on their back with a pillow for extra support is always a good idea in any case.

A Note of Caution: Please do not use any oil on the forehead. Avoid eye area with irritants. Thank you!

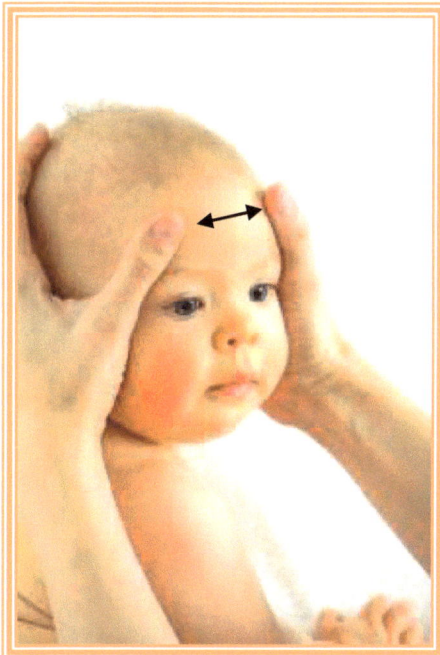

"Fulling the Forehead"

This technique is the same principle as previous steps in fulling. This one starts in the middle of the forehead, and slowly moves with all four fingers towards the outer temples.

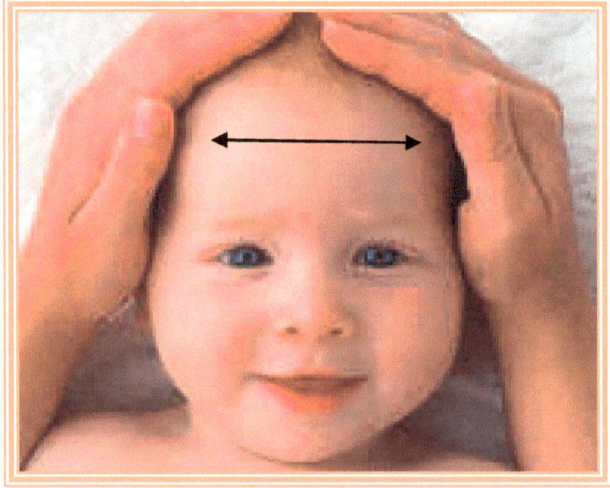

Note: Please avoid direct contact with the eyes while applying facial massage to your baby. If baby fusses, just move to another area of the body, and continue face later.

"Massaging the Temples"

1) Baby sits, facing away from you while you massage the temples.

2) This is a very simple technique. Apply soft, upward, circular motion at the temples. Next to the end of the eyebrow you will find a natural indentation. Avoid the eye area with your fingers, and if baby is not holding still, discontinue to avoid injury to eyes.

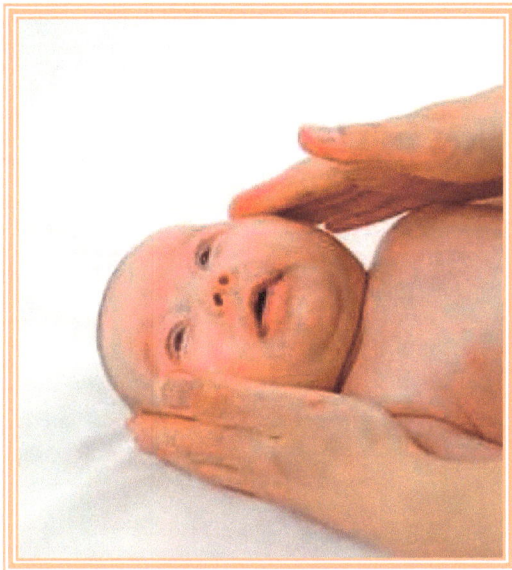

This massage can be done when baby is sleepy!

"Acupressure Ear Massage"

1) Rotation while holding the ear lobe with your index finger and thumb

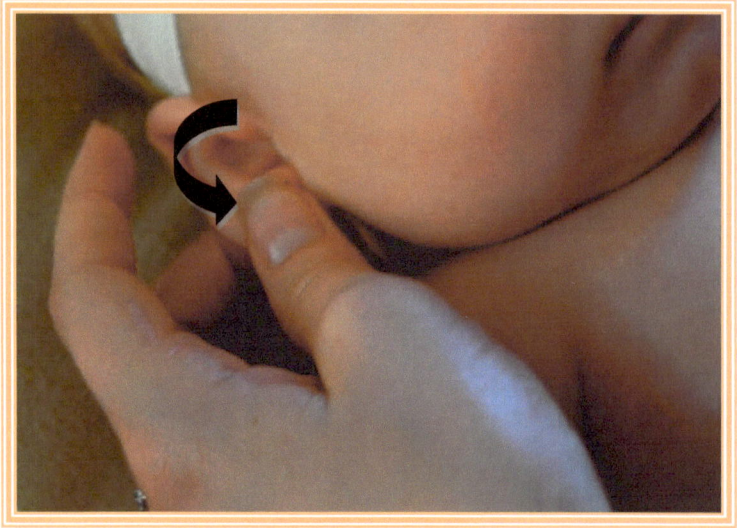

Note: This massage movement is done delicately, so the ear only moves slightly. If you baby doesn't care for this, then stick with the temple massage instead. Check with you doctor in the event of ear infections, or anything that might contraindicate the delica area of baby's ears.

"Acupressure Ear Massage" Cont.

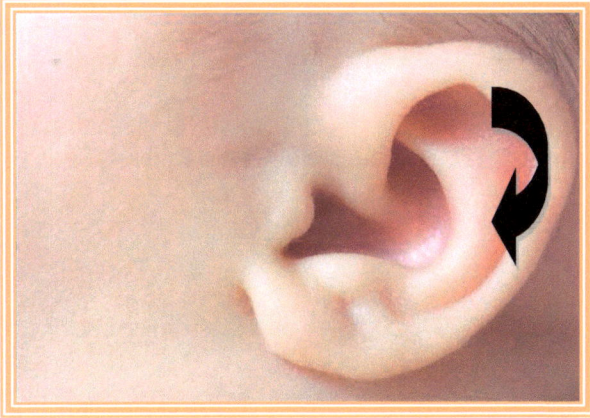

ote: Ear massage feels great when a baby is trying to get over an ear infection. It lps to bring circulation into the tissue area, and clears the inflammation.

"Foot Massage"

This massage for the feet feels sooo gooood!

1) Apply very light pressure on the foot (thumbs work great for this).

2) Fulling: Start at the middle and top of the foot, and smoothly move hand outward (like fulling for the stomach/tummy). (Refer to fulling basics.)

3) Kneading: The foot with a closed knuckle — it is a bit like working a baker' dough!

4) Tapotement: Light, gentle tapping with your fingertips, like playing the piano

5) Energy strokes should be done several times. Start from the top working you way to the bottom of the foot, using an open palm, barely touching the skin. kinda tickles! Gently apply.

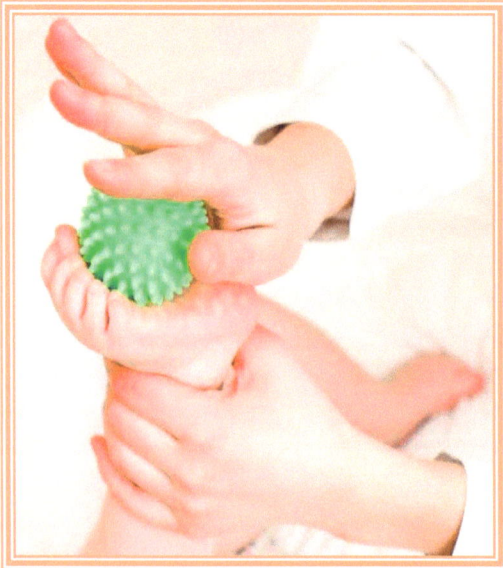

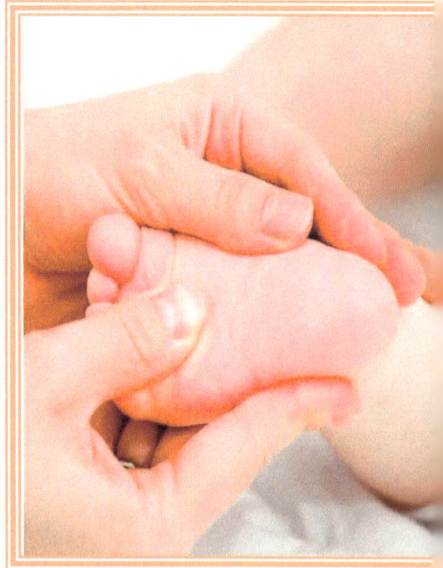

"Acupressure for Baby's Feet"

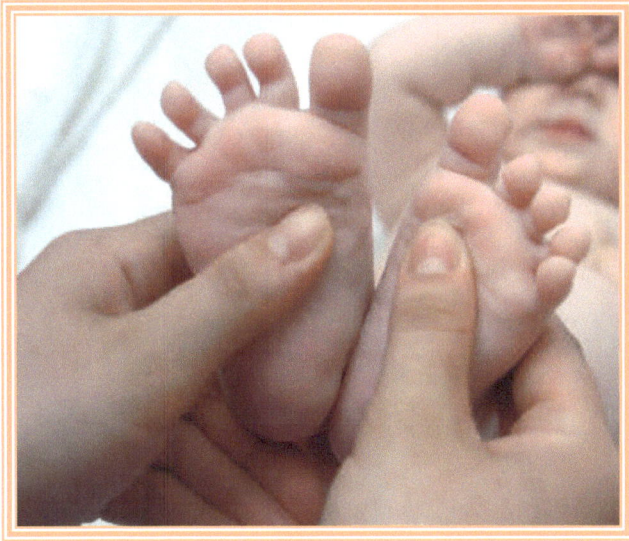

Pushen - Acupressure point at back of ankle: Use for crying fits, coma, and convulsions.

Yongquan - The sole of the foot: use for reducing fever, heat, vomiting, chest stiffness, urination problems, and general irritability.

Pushen - acupressure points Yongquan acupressure point Acupressure for Baby's Feet.

Foot Massage feels so good!

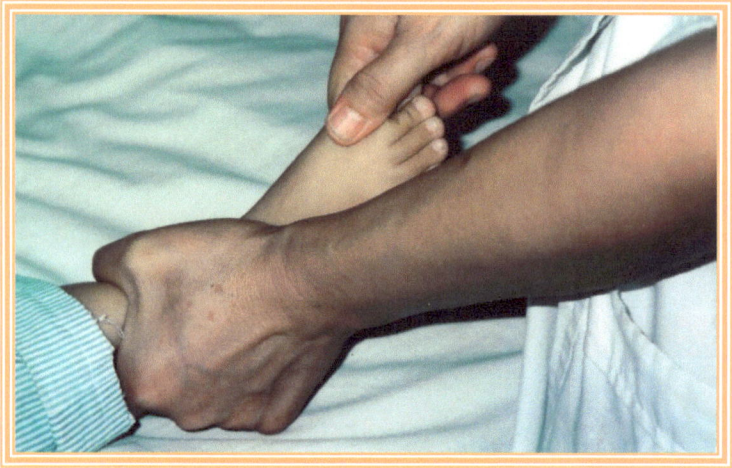

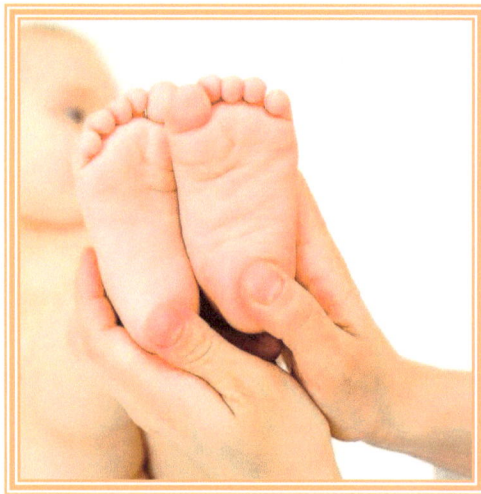

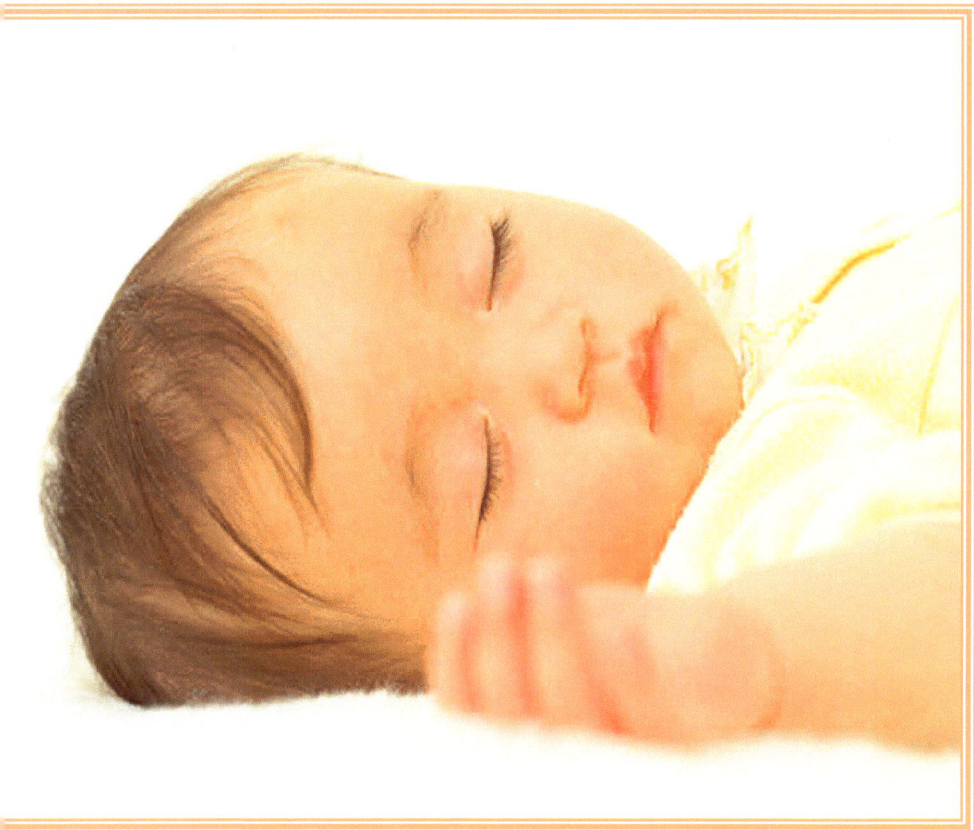

Sweet Dreams… after your Baby's Massage!

Acupressure for Baby

Note: The acupressure points listed here are the most commonly used in baby massage. Not all of th *explanation for use of acupressure points are listed here, only those points that are safe for hom* *application. For further references, see your local Acupuncturist or Chinese Medicine Doctor.*

Acupressure for the Front of Baby's Body

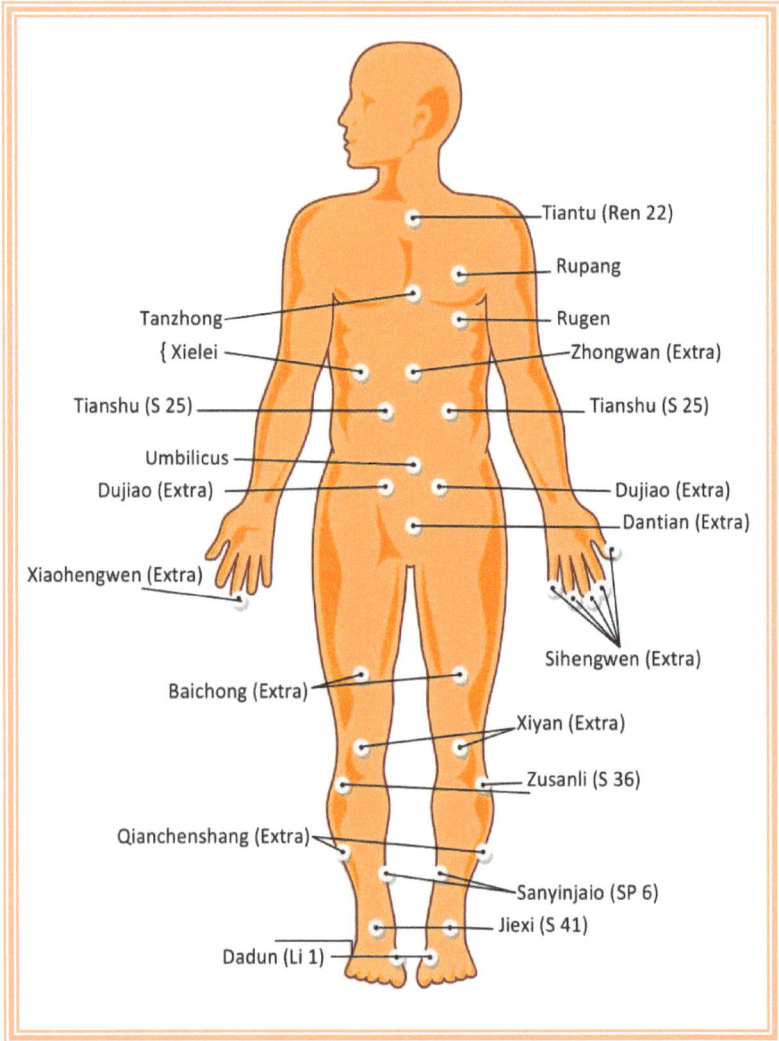

Tiantu (Ren 22)
Rupang
Rugen
Tanzhong
{ Xielei
Zhongwan (Extra)
Tianshu (S 25)
Tianshu (S 25)
Umbilicus
Dujiao (Extra)
Dujiao (Extra)
Dantian (Extra)
Xiaohengwen (Extra)
Sihengwen (Extra)
Baichong (Extra)
Xiyan (Extra)
Zusanli (S 36)
Qianchenshang (Extra)
Sanyinjiao (SP 6)
Jiexi (S 41)
Dadun (Li 1)

Commonly used "Tuina" points on the front

49

Acupressure for Baby's Chest

Tiantu — Lower throat suprasternum fossa; for congestion Relief

Shanzhong — Middle of sternum; for coughing, stuffy chest, asthma, vomiting and nausea

Rugen — Below nipple front of body; for lungs, cough and phlegm

Xielei — Below intercostal rib areas; relief of abdominal chest accumulation of phlegm

Acupressure for Baby's Stomach

Fuyinyang — Upper abdomen; for stomach, spleen and digestive relief

Zhongwan — Middle of stomach; for stomach, spleen and digestive relief

Duqi — Navel area; for abdominal digestion

Dantian — Middle of lower abdomen; for strengthening the kidneys, digestive relief and hernia

Dujiao — Below belly button; for digestive relief and Diarrhea

Tianshu — 2 thumbs lateral from the belly button; for movement of food, constipation, indigestion and digestive relief

Acupressure for Baby's Face

Zanzhu (or Tianting) — Middle of eyebrow, soothing nerves and headach relief

Tiayang — Sides of eyebrows, removing heat, eyes and relief from pain

Yingxiang — Near nostrils, reducing fever

Yanguan (or Jiache) — Lower mandible, facial trauma, paralysis, an mouth opening

Renzhong — The point of great balance, for dizzy spells, and trauma

Ermen (or Fengmen) — Mouth opening at mandible for toothache, paralys of face, convulsions, tinnitus and deafness.

Chengjiang — start at center of the chin and massage towards jaw Yanguan acupressure point. Can be used for tightness in the jaw, faci paralyisis, and relief from inflammation during ear infections.

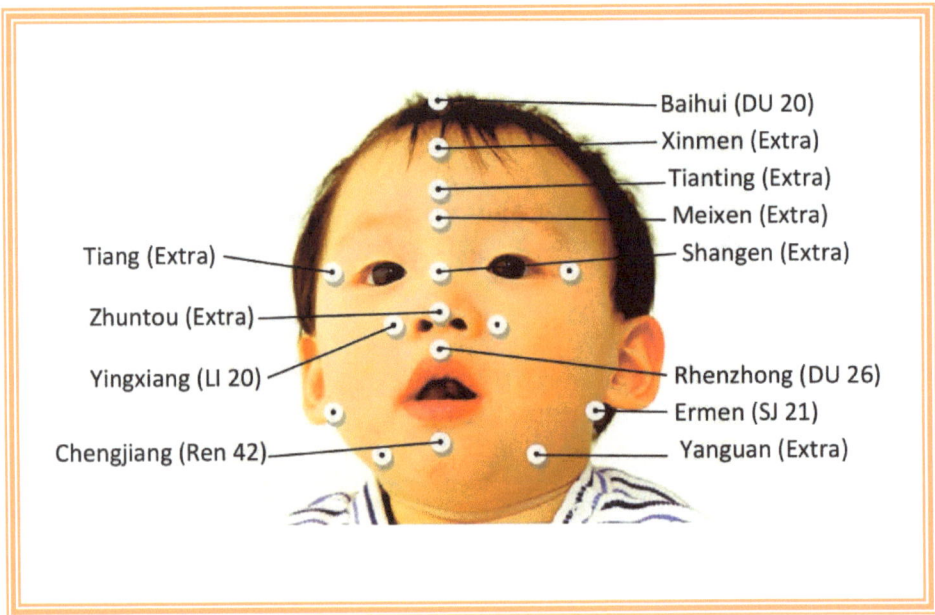

Acupressure for Baby's Face

Zhuntou — Massage upward from tip of nose towards forehead to Shangen,

Meixen, Tianting, Xinmen to Baihu (top of head). See below for massaging

Xinmen. Can be used for soothing nerves, headache relief, blurred vision and nasal congestion relief.

Massaging Xinmen — Lightly stroke forehead from middle of forehead to eyebrows to the top of forehead to hair.

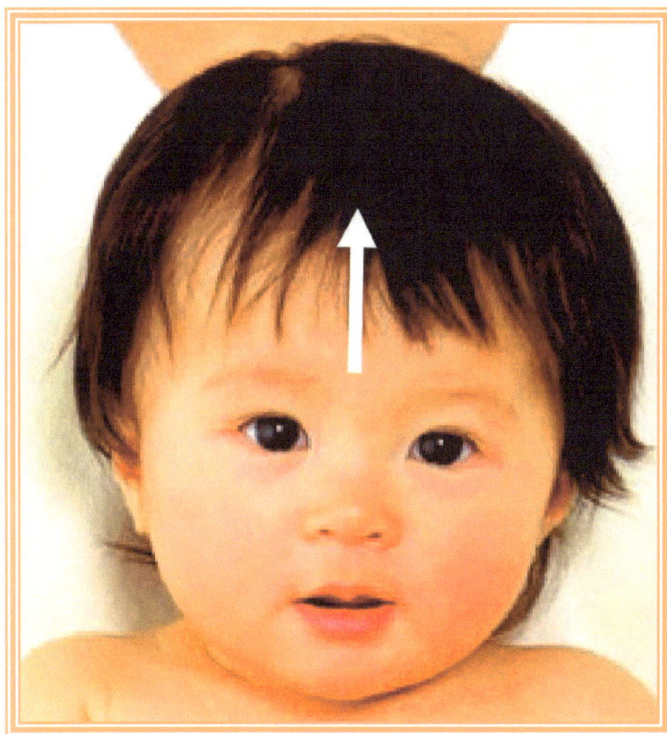

Note: This Chinese Acupressure technique may relieve convulsions, spasm, tension of eyes, blurry vision, dizziness and nasal congestion.

Acupressure for Baby's Back

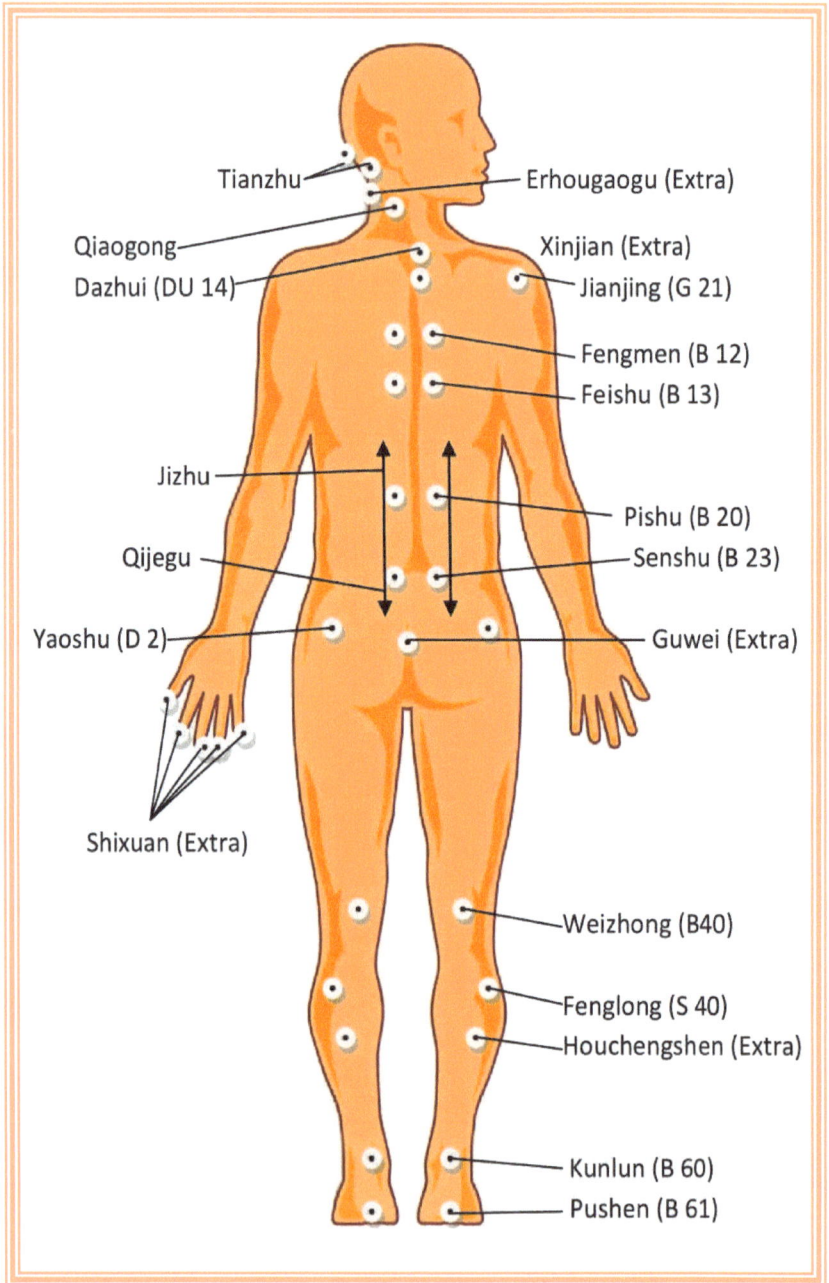

Tianzhu
Qiaogong
Dazhui (DU 14)
Jizhu
Qijegu
Yaoshu (D 2)
Shixuan (Extra)

Erhougaogu (Extra)
Xinjian (Extra)
Jianjing (G 21)
Fengmen (B 12)
Feishu (B 13)
Pishu (B 20)
Senshu (B 23)
Guwei (Extra)
Weizhong (B40)
Fenglong (S 40)
Houchengshen (Extra)
Kunlun (B 60)
Pushen (B 61)

Acupressure for Baby's Back

Jizhu — Lumbosacral region on back; for soothing the central nervous system, malnutrition, diarrhea, vomiting, abdominal pains and constipation

Pishu — 11th thoracic vertebrae on back; helping function of spleen, digestion, and chronic weakness

Qijiegu — 4th lumbar vertebrae on back; for diarrhea, dysentery, prolapsed rectum and constipation

Guiwei — Tip of coccyx on back; diarrhea, dysentery, abdominal pain, and prolapsed rectum

Changqiang — Tip of coccyx; for intestinal inflammation

Acupressure for Baby's Neck and Shoulder

Qiaogong — Side of neck; for rigidity, stiffness, and pain in the neck area

Erhougaogu — Behind ear; for restlessness, calming and congestion of the head

Xinjian — 2nd and 3rd cervical vertebrae; clearing the throat, helps congestion, sort throat and heat

Tianzhu — Hairline at back of neck; for stiff neck and common cold headaches

Dazhui — 7th cervical vertebrae at back of neck; for heat, common cold, fever and vomiting

Feishu — 3rd thoracic vertebrae on back; for lungs, relief from coughing and asthma

Acupressure for Baby's Arm and Hand (Palm)

Sanguan—The radial border of forearm; for digestive relief, cold weak arms

Tianeshui—The medial border of forearm; for fever, cold relief and irritability

Liufu—Ulnar side of forearm; Cooling the body during heat spells, detoxificatio and clearing heat which the body stores

Neibagua—Around in a circle in the palm of the hand, rotate gently clockwis harmonizing the cough, diarrhea, abdomen, digestive pains, food digestion, a abdominal pain relief

Dahengwen—On the wrist crease, palm up; Press the point gently with bo thumbs and do fulling to outer wrist. Can relieve vomiting, chills, fever, asthm spitting up, food stagnation, abdominal distension, and diarrhea

Zongjin—Mid point of the wrist crease on the palm; Knead with thumb gently 15 20 times, clockwise. Can be used for convulsions, mental stress, diarrhe vomiting and mouth ulcers

Yujijiao—Middle end of wrist crease on the palm; Tap the point lightly 7 to 8 tim with pointer finger. Can be used for stopping convulsions, easing the min brightening the eyes, clearing pathogenic heat, epilepsy, blurred vision, rednes pain and swelling of the eye, excessive crying

Banmen—The second phalangeal joint of the thumb near Yuji; Hold, rub the poi with thumb gently clockwise 75 to 100 times. Can be used for acute or chror convulsions and indigestion

Neilaogong—In the center of the palm; Knead gently clock-wise 30-75 times. C be used for convulsions caused by fright, reducing fever of common cold, a excessive heat

Pijing—The radial side of the thumb between the tip and the base of the thumb. reinforce spleen (can be used for constipation), stroke towards the heart 100 tim and for reducing (can be used for diarrhea) stroke away from the heart 100 times

Xinjing—The tip of the middle finger. Stroke towards the heart for reinforci (diarrhea relief) and away from the heart for reducing (constipation relief)

Feijing—Tip of ring finger; Hold point for 30 seconds. Can be used for comm cold, cough, asthma, spitting up and constipation

Acupressure for Baby's Arm and Hand (Palm) cont'd

Shending—The tip of the littlest finger; Knead the tip gently 75 to 100 times. Can be used for night sweats.

Yunshuirutu to Yunturushui—From tip of little finger forming a half circle all the way to the base of the thumb (see diagram, page 40). For dysuria, yellow urine, and constipation.

Hongchi—Crease of the forearm; Guide fingers gently from Hongchi up to Tianshui at the crease of wrist to Zhongjian. Can be used for fever, cold, mental stress, external cold.

Tuichi—Gently stroking Liufu (6 Fu organs) away from heart towards wrist. Can be used for fever, cold, restlessness, irritability.

Sanguan—Stroke gently; Radial border of forearm between crease in arm all the way to crease in wrist. Can be used to strengthen Yang energy or treat exterior (common cold) cold symptoms from pathogenic factors.

Acupressure for Baby's Hand & Arm (Back of Hand)

Yiwofeng—The depression of the middle of the wrist at the crease (top of baby's wrist); press the point with index finger or thumb about 75 to 100 times for warming the middle jiao, promoting circulation of qi, relieving abdominal pain, and stop-ping joint pain.

Weiling—The top of the hand between second and third metacarpal bones, beside the Wailaogong point; press the point 2 to 5 times with the tip of thumb, then gently rub after pressing. This point can resuscitate from coma, and is good for tinnitus, headache, and unconsciousness caused by acute convulsions.

Jingning—On the top of hand beside Wailaogong point between the fourth and fifth metacarpal bones. Press the point with thumb 2 to 5 times, and then gently knead for about ten seconds; May help with asthma and excessive spitting up, palpating the lumps in the abdomen or gassy full stomach and chest area.

Wailaogong—In the center (of the top) of the hand opposite Neilaogong point. Knead the point for three to five minutes gently; can be used for warming the yang energy of the body, diarrhea, dysentery from common cold, prolapsed rectum, ascariasis, hernia, and borborygmia.

Eryangchi—Stroke gently towards wrist from anterior middle of the forearm. Can be good for promoting circulation and digestive relief

Acupressure for Baby's Hand & Arm (Back of Hand), cont'd

Ershanmen—In the center of the top of the hand in the de-pression between the third and fourth metacarpal bones. Press the point 3 to 5 times gently; Can be used for promoting better circulation of blood and relaxing tendons and good for asthma, cold from wind, stiffness in the chest, spit-ting up, and clearing the common cold symptoms.

Laolong—The tip of the middle finger. Press 3 to 7 times; Can help to resuscitate an unconscious baby, stop convulsions, reduce fever, an pathogenic fire qi (excessive heat).

Duanzheng—At the middle finger nail root (base of nail). Press sides of baby's middle finger with thumb and index finger (as to squeeze) 3 to times; can help with dysentery, diarrhea, vomiting, and spastic colon.

Erma—On the top of the hand in the depression between the ring finger and the little finger. Hold and gently rub the point with thumb up to 2 times; can be used for reinforcing the yin energy of qi in the body, dysuria indigestion, pro-lapsed rectum, abdominal pain, weak body constitution cough, asthma, and difficulty expelling toxins.

Tianmenruhukou—Between thumb and index finger (top of hand). Press point up to 75 times; can be used for smoothing circulation, clenched teeth, sore throat, fullness in the chest.

Wuzhijie—On the top of hand of all five fingers phalang-ometacarpal joints Press points 3 to 5 times; can help with resuscitating an unconscious baby, stopping convulsions, and calming the baby.

Shixuan—All five tips of fingers. Press points 1 to 3 times; can be good for resuscitating unconscious baby, acute convulsions, dull behavior, and crying fits.

Acupressure for Baby's Arm and Hand (Palm)

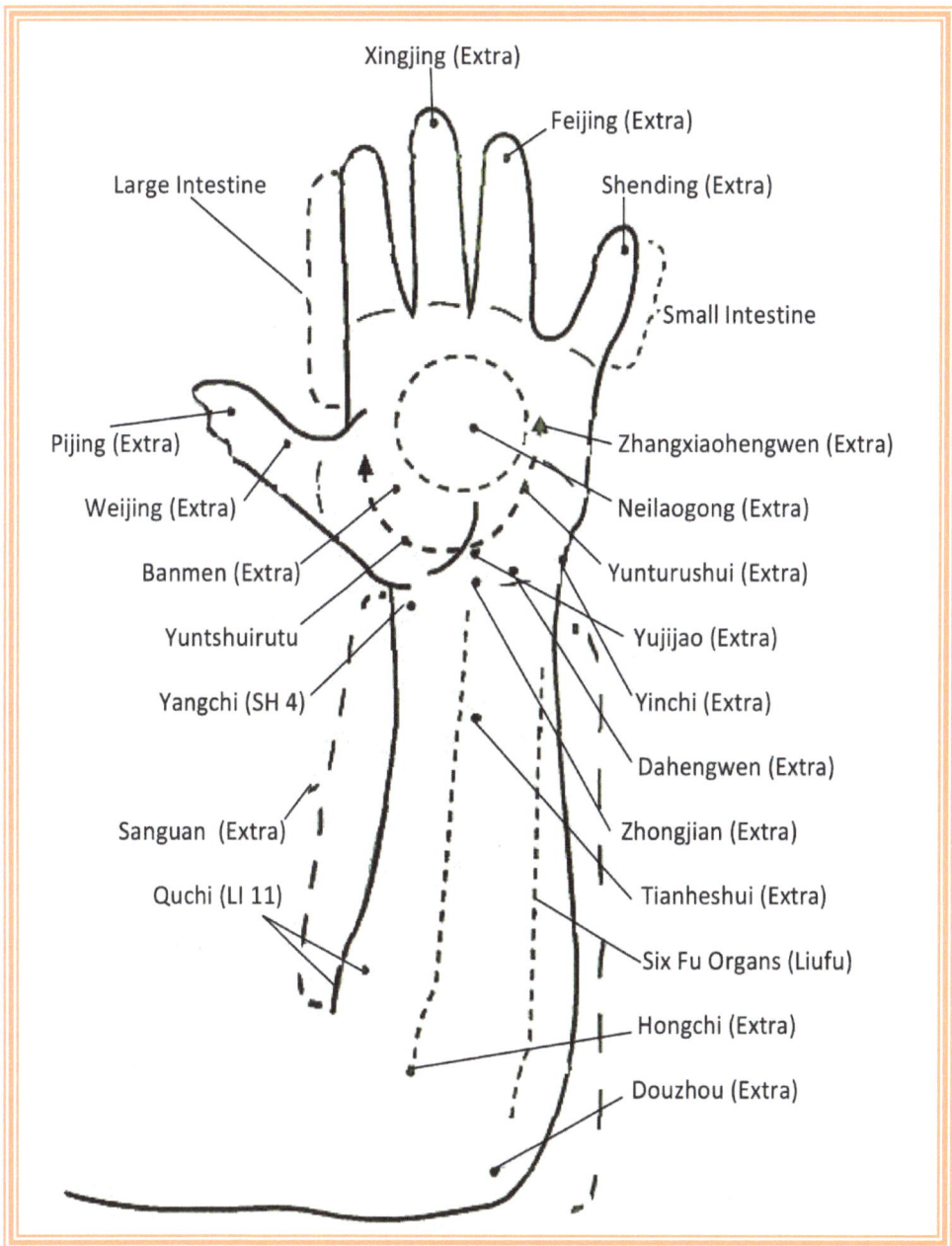

Xingjing (Extra)

Feijing (Extra)

Large Intestine

Shending (Extra)

Small Intestine

Pijing (Extra)

Zhangxiaohengwen (Extra)

Weijing (Extra)

Neilaogong (Extra)

Banmen (Extra)

Yunturushui (Extra)

Yuntshuirutu

Yujijao (Extra)

Yangchi (SH 4)

Yinchi (Extra)

Dahengwen (Extra)

Sanguan (Extra)

Zhongjian (Extra)

Quchi (LI 11)

Tianheshui (Extra)

Six Fu Organs (Liufu)

Hongchi (Extra)

Douzhou (Extra)

Acupressure for Baby's Hand & Arm (Back of Hand)

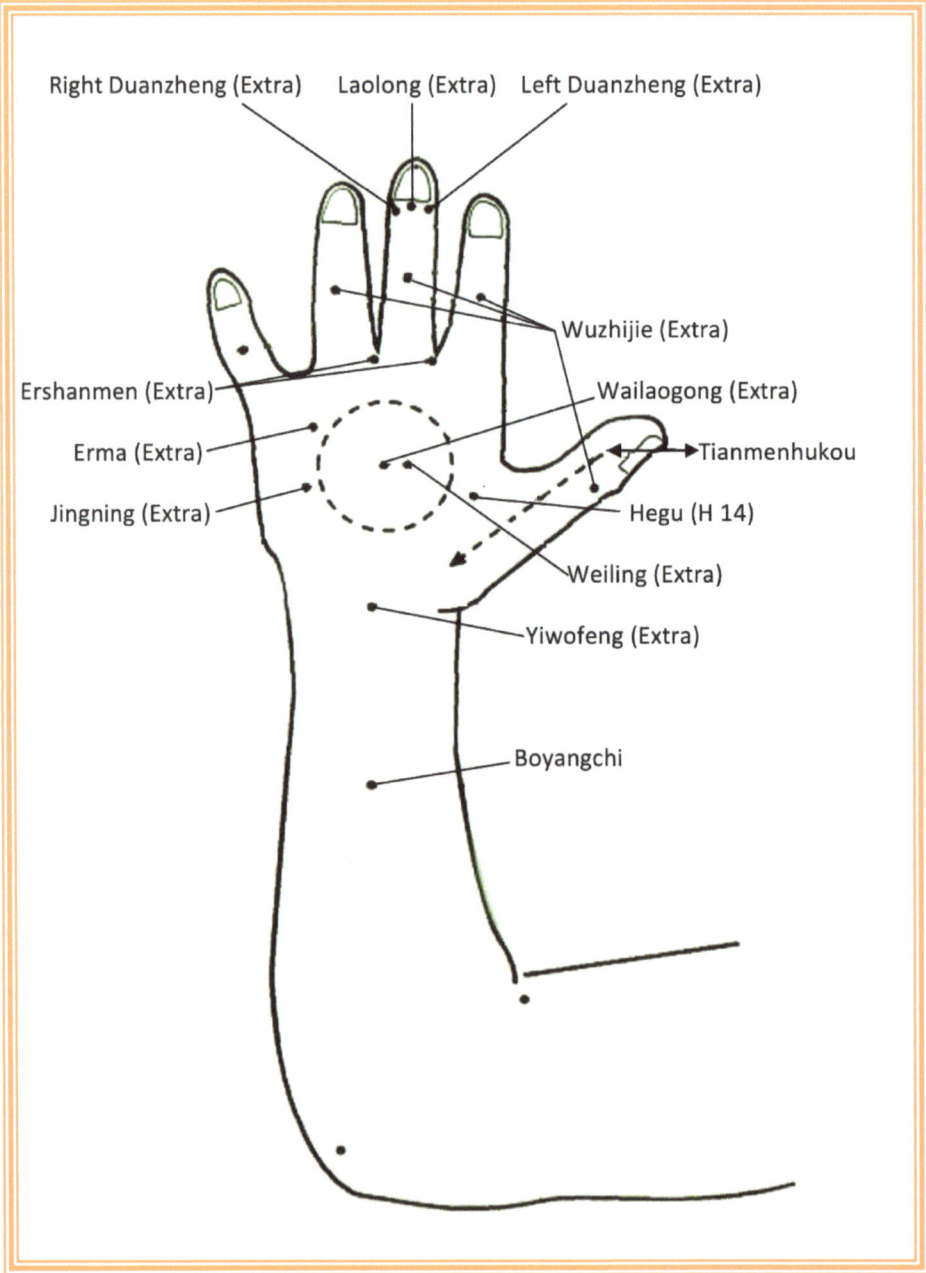

Right Duanzheng (Extra)   Laolong (Extra)   Left Duanzheng (Extra)

Wuzhijie (Extra)

Ershanmen (Extra)

Wailaogong (Extra)

Erma (Extra)

Tianmenhukou

Jingning (Extra)

Hegu (H 14)

Weiling (Extra)

Yiwofeng (Extra)

Boyangchi

References and Resources

Hippocrates, 400 B.C. Hippocrates has been a valuable resource and scholar light years ahead of his time, some 400 B.C. ahead of his time. His insight and knowledge forever live on in textbooks across the world, and may be found in any library whilst looking for your favorite books and authors although Hippocrates has no original book published in his name.

Andre Virel, French Psychoanalyst. The information that Andre Virel has imparted through his brilliant work with his patients in psychotherapy on how aromatherapy works with the limbic (emotional part of the brain) system in the human body.

Health and Nutritional support: La Leche League. This company provides support to all new mothers and care-givers to new babies. There is a national informational line you can call, and connect with other mothers and ask common questions and concerns about being a new mother. Look in your local telephone directory on how to contact the La Leche League.

Mannatech Inc. For optimal health during pregnancy, immune support, advanced weight-loss system after pregnancy, learning about safe neutraceutical (proven non-toxic) health products. Jammie is an Independent sales and marketing representative for Mannatech, Inc. This company offers a source for innovative and advanced natural products for breast feeding nutrition, immune system, chronic fatigue, candidiasis and general nutritional needs. The American Naturopathic Medical Association has presented its highest scientific honor of recognition for the development of the nutritional carbohydrate complex, Mannatech's Ambrotose®, which was awarded "The Most Significant Progress Made in Biochemistry" for 1996. In addition, some new studies with Mannatech have shown that children with ADD and ADHD have been helped by Mannatech's Ambrotose®. For more information on Mannatech, Inc. contact www.Mannatech.com

PEPS - An early parenthood support system, and may be found in your local area. The PEPS groups offer support systems for most common asked questions when you are a new parent. For more information on PEPS, look in your local telephone directory. New parent groups will often meet in the home, and locations are supported nationally throughout the medical clinics and hospitals.

Planned Parenthood - A service provided for educational purposes, can be found in your local telephone directory. Each local Planned Parenthood group offers classes on birthing, doula, infant massage, breast feeding, health planning, and medical care for those who are planning to become or already are new parents.

Beinfield, H. & Korngold, E. (1991) Between Heaven and Earth: A Guide to Chinese Medicine. Harriet Beinfield, L.Ac. and Efrein Korngold, L.Ac., O.M.D. are co-authors of this book. "Worthy and important...this book will be a valuable source for all those interested in combining the best of the East and West," Deepok Chopra, M.D., author of Ageless Body, Timeless Mind. Toronto, Canada: Random House.

McDougall, John & Mary (1999). The McDougall Program for Women. This book contain information on nutrition, food recipes by Mary McDougall, heart disease, cancer, diabetes, stress depression, and many other vital medical issues confronting women today. John McDougal M.D., Mary his wife and family have a medical practice and reside in Santa Rosa, CA. Origina work published in N.Y., N.Y.: Dutton, a member of Penguin Putnam, Inc.

Robbins, J. (1996). Reclaiming Your Health: Exploding the Medical Myth and Embracing th Source of True Healing. John Robbins (author of Diet for a New America). This book include information from the world's leading experts on the dietary link to the environment and healt John Robbins is the founder of Earth Save, Intl., a non-profit organization that supports health food choices, preservation of the environment, and a more compassionate world. John Robbir lives with his family in Santa Cruz, CA. Published by H.J. Kramer, Inc. in Tiburon, CA.

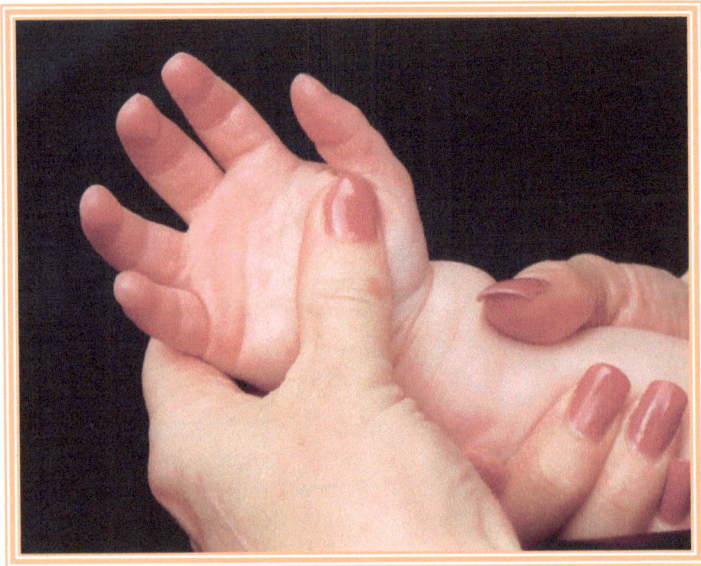

"Neibagua Massage - Around and around in a circle, rotating clockwise, the palm of your hand, the center of the universe."

About the Author

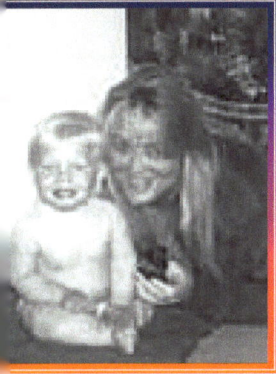

Linda Larson shares delightful baby massage techniques from all around the world, and continues to write and publish children's Fairytales, and a recipe cook book all good Fairies will enjoy in the kitchen with their extended Spriten spirit family members and friends. Linda is an alchemist in the kitchen while concocting very tasty Quinoa Fusion Recipes and Gourmet Cooking tips with her readers and fans while introducing them to the world of healthy food alternatives for energetic lifestyles. Although, she spends a great deal of time writing and publishing, her most important priority is her love of sharing joy-filled Fairytale stories, cook books and whole food cooking methods with people around the world.

Linda is excited to share the promotion of easy to cook meals incorporating Quinoa – The Ancient Grain of the Aztecs, a healthy gourmet lifestyle and has over 23 Certifications in the profession of Ancient Healing Arts to locations such as; China, Japan, Turkey, U.K. and Ireland. Her Culinary Healing Arts endeavors have far reached around the world to many people's families, friends and children with a vision to assist the healing of each person's body, mind, spirit and to be fun inspired where these products are meant to also excite the palate.

Body, Mind & Spirit: Linda studies and practices meditation and prayer. She loves art, music, movies, whole foods, Fairytale stories, all animals, horseback riding, organic farming, agriculture, gourmet cooking, creating yummy recipes and extraordinary culinary adventures.

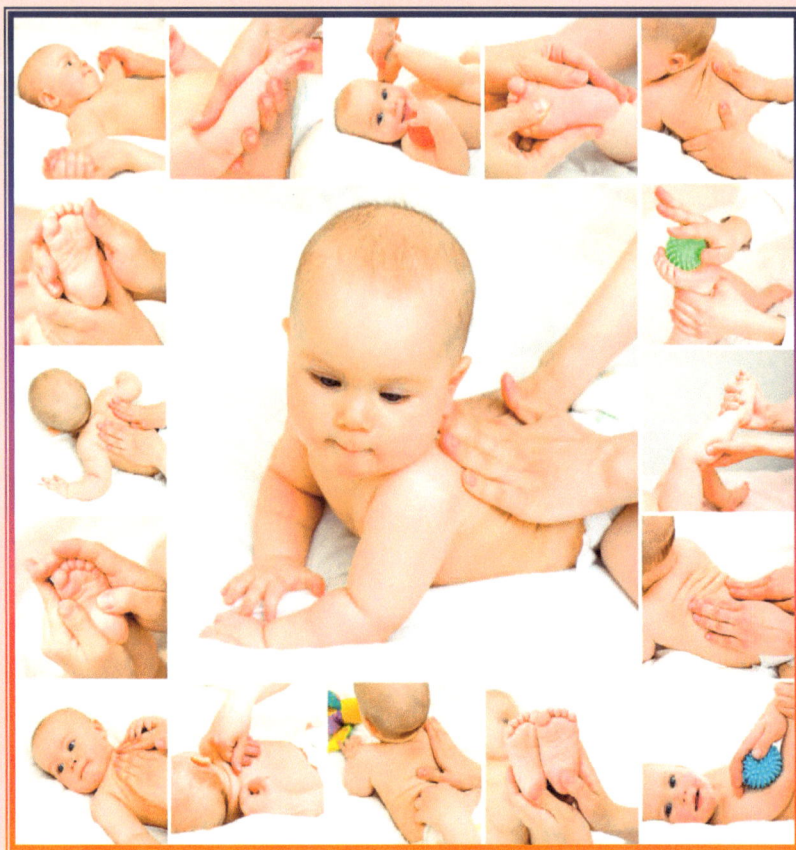

"TUINA Baby Massage" A great gift at a baby shower for an expecting Moth Massage Therapy is a delight for babies. There is pain relief with colic, common cold a flu just to name a few. Human Touch to the neuroreceptors sends signals through the sp or central nervous system. After the brain answers the telephone call from neurotransmitter, it begins to produce liver proteins; scientifically described to help w building better memory and brain function. This then triggers hormones through pituitary gland. Endorphins, which are our natural pain relievers, are produced a released from the pituitary. Another important factor is the increased AC (Adrenocorticotrophic Hormone) levels ultimately produced through our pituitary gla directly affecting the function of the adrenals. A secretion of hormones begins to mo directly into the immune system. Lymphatic stimulus (the immune system glands) then occur, which is good for your baby's health! Enjoy "Baby Massage Delight" - A us friendly guide to developing a life-long bond of joy, health and well-being.